FUNDAMENTALS OF
# Orthopaedic Biomechanics

# FUNDAMENTALS OF

# Orthopaedic Biomechanics

## ALBERT H. BURSTEIN, PH.D.

Senior Scientist
Department of Biomechanics
Hospital for Special Surgery
New York, New York

## TIMOTHY M. WRIGHT, PH.D.

Director
Department of Biomechanics
Hospital for Special Surgery
New York, New York

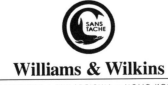

**Williams & Wilkins**

BALTIMORE • PHILADELPHIA • HONG KONG
LONDON • MUNICH • SYDNEY • TOKYO

A WAVERLY COMPANY

*Editor:* William M. Passano III
*Project Manager:* Raymond E. Reter
*Copy Editor:* David Mason, Publication Services, Inc.
*Designer:* Jim Proefrock, Publication Services, Inc.
*Original Artwork:* Mollie Dunker and Jacqueline Schaffer
*Cover Designer:* Jim Proefrock, Publication Services, Inc.

Copyright ©1994
Williams & Wilkins
428 East Preston Street
Baltimore, Maryland 21202 U.S.A.

Accurate indications, adverse reactions, and dosage schedules for drugs are provided in this book, but it is possible that they may change. The reader is urged to review the package information data of the manufacturers of the medications mentioned.

*Printed in the United States of America.*

Chapter reprints are available from the publisher.

**Library of Congress Cataloging-in-Publication Data**
Burstein, Albert H.
    Fundamentals of orthopaedic biomechanics / Albert H. Burstein,
Timothy M. Wright.
      p.    cm.
    Includes bibliographical references and index.
    ISBN 0-683-01135-9
    1. Musculoskeletal system–Mechanical properties.   2. Orthopedic
implants–Mechanical properties.    3. Orthopedic surgery.
I. Wright, Timothy M.  II. Title.  III. Title: Orthopaedic
biomechanics.
    [DNLM: 1. Biomechanics.    WE   103 B972f  1994]
RD732.B87    1994
612.7′6–dc20
DNLM/DLC
for Library of Congress                                        93-45784
                                                CIP
                                    94 95 96 97
1 2 3 4 5 6 7 8 9 10

*To Myra and Kathy*

# Foreword

The authors have written an immensely practical book on biomechanics. This should be an important resource for anyone concerned with the supporting and locomotor functions of the body or in various aspects of state-of-the-art reparative or reconstructive bone and joint surgery. For students of orthopaedic surgery, physical medicine and rehabilitation, or biomechanics it should become an essential introductory text.

The tremendous advances of orthopaedic surgery during the past 30 years owe much to the post–World War II marriage of the interests of mechanical engineering scientists with those of orthopaedic surgeons. This book is a natural issue of that marriage. It is written by two influential experts who have devoted their professional lives to the development of biomechanical science and who have tirelessly contributed to the promotion of its intimate interaction with orthopaedic surgery through their research, developmental work, and teaching.

This book clearly explains the current state of the science, not only through textual description but also by clear graphs, diagrams, and relatively simple and understandable equations.

The book is organized into seven chapters, carrying the reader through forces and moments in the musculoskeletal system, musculoskeletal performance, joint stability, mechanical behavior of materials, mechanical behavior of bone, and performance of orthopaedic implant systems.

Each chapter is subindexed and titled so that the book can easily be used as a reference resource and for review purposes. Each chapter also provides a short list of references for the reader who wants to explore a subject to a greater depth.

In their preface, the authors state that their goal is to present engineering principles for determining biomechanical factors influencing treatment choices. My review of the text indicates very clearly that they have achieved their goal. A knowlege of the material presented in this book is essential for the up-to-date practice of orthopaedic surgery. Every orthopaedic surgeon and most other professionals concerned with the management of patients with musculoskeletal conditions, no matter what their etiology or origin, should have this text close at hand. I certainly will.

Philip D. Wilson, Jr., M.D.
Surgeon-in-Chief Emeritus
The Hospital for Special Surgery

# Preface

Biomechanics is the study of the effect of forces on biological systems. In orthopaedics and related fields of study, the biological system of interest is the musculoskeletal system. Our intention, then, is to use this book as a vehicle to teach the orthopaedist, resident, physical therapist, and other health professional the way in which the musculoskeletal system, and the implants that are used to replace or support it, are affected by forces. These are the forces encountered in everyday activities and trauma.

Our goal in writing this book was to present engineering principles that should provide the reader with the skills necessary for determining biomechanical factors that will influence treatment choices. Emphasis is on basic mechanical principles, and mathematics is limited to basic algebra. Biomaterials are discussed in terms of the influences of material properties on mechanical behavior. We did not intend this book to be a thorough analytical treatment of engineering principles or an exhaustive treatment of biomaterials. We are presenting first principles, and we leave it to the reader to seek advanced textbooks when so motivated. References are kept to a minimum and are used primarily to support specific examples in the text.

The authors would like to acknowledge the assistance of Leonor Troyano in typing the manuscript, Mollie Dunker and Jacqi Schaffer in preparing the artwork, and their colleagues in the Department of Biomechanics at the Hospital for Special Surgery who have collaborated in developing some of the examples included in this book.

*Longboat Key, Florida*                                        Albert H. Burstein

*Stamford, Connecticut*                                      Timothy M. Wright

# Contents

# 1

## Forces and Moments in the Musculoskeletal System

**FORCES AND MOMENTS**

**STATIC EQUILIBRIUM**

**PROBLEMS SOLVED ASSUMING STATIC EQUILIBRIUM**

**DYNAMIC EQUILIBRIUM**

## FORCES AND MOMENTS

*Forces* and *moments* affect the way in which all body segments move. The tendency for any type of motion can be explained in terms of these two concepts.

### Force

*A force is defined as that quantity that tends to change the velocity (to accelerate) an object.* The magnitude of the force is related to the resulting acceleration by one of Sir Isaac Newton's laws of motion, which states that the magnitude of the force is equal to the mass of the object being accelerated, multiplied by the resulting acceleration of the object:

$$\text{Force} = \text{Mass} \times \text{Acceleration} \tag{1.1}$$

A force applied to an object can therefore cause the object to move faster or slower. A force can also cause an object to change its direction of motion. Thus, if an object is acted upon by a force that constantly changes direction, the object will follow a curved path.

Standards have been established to define the unit of measure of all basic physical quantities such as force. For example, the standard international system of weights and measures has established the kilogram as the unit of mass. Note that this is the only standard quantity that is not a unit quantity, since a kilogram (kg) is equal to 1000 grams. The international unit for distance is the meter (m) and for time is the second (sec). Thus, the units of force are the units of mass (kg) multiplied by the units of acceleration $(m/sec^2)$. The resulting unit of force $(kg \cdot m/sec^2)$ is called a newton (N).

The newton is also a unit of weight. Weight is the force of gravity attempting to accelerate an object toward the center of the earth. A freely falling object under the influence of gravity will increase its velocity (that is, it will accelerate) at a constant rate of 9.8 meters per second per second. A patient with a mass of 70 kilograms, for example, has a weight of 686 newtons:

$$\text{Weight} = \text{Mass} \times \text{Acceleration}$$

$$= 70 \text{ kg} \times 9.8 \text{ m/sec}^2$$

$$= 686 \text{ N}$$

If the patient is unrestrained, the patient's mass would be accelerated toward the center of the earth at 9.8 meters per $second^2$. Similarly, a total knee femoral component made from cobalt alloy that weighs 4 newtons has a mass of 0.4 kilograms. If the component slips out of your hand, it accelerates to the floor (toward the center of the earth) at 9.8 meters/$second^2$. And a 10-pound (44-newton) weight applied to a leg in traction has a mass of 4.5 kilograms. If the traction rope breaks, the 4.5-kilogram mass would accelerate toward the floor, increasing its velocity 9.8 meters per second for every second it fell.

## Moment

*A moment is defined as that quantity that tends to change the angular velocity of an object.* For example, when a power reamer is used in the operating room, the angular velocity at which the reamer turns can be increased only by applying a moment (or torque) to the reamer. In fact, as the angular velocity increases, the surgeon has to provide a resisting torque to keep the reamer from spinning out of his or her hand. Similar to the action of a force, a moment tends to angularly accelerate an object in a manner proportional to a quantity related to the mass of the object. The concept of a more massive object requiring a larger force to cause the same straight-line acceleration is straightforward. The concept for changing angular velocity is similar, but not identical. *The proportional constant between the moment applied to an object and the resulting angular acceleration is the mass moment of inertia:*

$$\text{Moment} = \text{Mass moment of inertia} \times \text{Angular acceleration} \qquad (1.2)$$

The mass moment of inertia depends not only on the mass of the object, but also on the distribution of the mass. For example, a tightrope walker can more effectively balance on the rope by extending his arms (Fig. 1.1). He has not changed his mass; he has merely changed the way in which his mass is distributed about his body. By moving the mass of his arms further from his body, he increases his mass moment of inertia. He can increase this effect by carrying a long, slender pole. The addition of the pole increases the total mass resting on the rope but, more importantly, distributes more mass further away from the center of his body. The effect of this redistribution is to allow him to minimize the angular accelerations his body will experience about the tightrope because of small moments caused by the misalignment of his center of mass over the rope.

In many situations involving conservative treatment of fractures, the physician can change both the amount of mass carried by a limb and the way that the mass is distributed. For example, in applying a cast to the leg, the physician can affect the mass of the cast by the choice of casting material and by the size of the cast. But the physician can also affect the mass moment of inertia of the cast (and, therefore, of the functional limb) by the location of the cast and, again, by its size. Affecting the mass moment of inertia, even without changing the mass of the cast, will affect the mechanics of moving the limb. As the mass moment of inertia of the limb is increased—for example, by applying the same cast farther down on the leg—the patient will need to exert larger moments to angularly accelerate the leg during gait.

The unit of mass moment of inertia is obtained by multiplying the mass of the object by the square of the distance between an equivalent location of the center of rotation of the object and an equivalent location of the center of mass. Suppose that the mass moment of inertia of the pole that the tightrope walker uses to help balance himself on the high wire is $5 \text{ kg} \cdot \text{m}^2$, as determined about his center of rotation (located directly above the rope). If he changed to

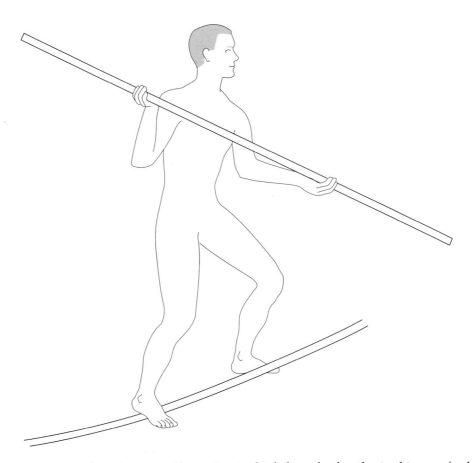

**Figure 1.1.** The tightrope walker maintains his balance by distributing his mass further away from the center of his body. He can easily do this by extending his arms or by having additional mass further away from the center of his body in the form of a pole. The pole increases his mass moment of inertia, thus preventing small moments (imbalance) from causing large angular displacements (falling).

a longer, more slender pole that had the same mass but was twice as long, the value of the mass moment of inertia would increase by a factor of 4 to 20 kg·m², giving him a much greater mass moment of inertia about the rope.

Since a moment is the product of the mass moment of inertia (kg · m²) and the angular acceleration (radians/sec²), the resulting unit of moment is kilogram-meters times meters/second² (kg · m²/sec²). (The unit of a radian is a ratio and therefore is dimensionless; see page 37.) But in the standard international system of weights and measures a newton is equal to 1 kilogram-meter/second², so the unit of moment is more commonly described as a newton-meter. For example, the manufacturer of an external fixation frame recommends that the nuts holding the frame together be tightened to a moment of 10 newton-meters. This moment can be created by manually applying a force of 50 newtons at the end of a 20-centimeter (0.2-meter) wrench (Fig. 1.2). It is common to produce moments in this way, by applying a force to a lever. Another method for creating a moment is to generate a couple, that is, a pair of equal and opposite forces acting at a distance about the center of rotation of the object to which the moment is to be applied. A screwdriver, for example, can be turned by the couple created by applying equal forces with two fingers placed directly opposite one another on the handle (Fig. 1.3).

Movements of the upper and lower extremities are created by moments generated about the joints. These moments are created both by external forces

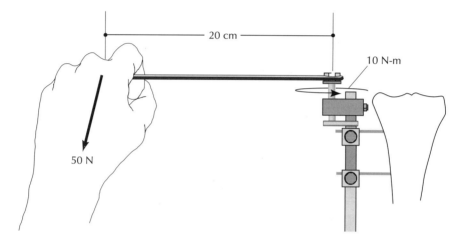

**Figure 1.2.** The application of a 50-newton force on the handle of the wrench at a distance of 20 centimeters from the nut on the external fixation frame creates a moment whose magnitude is 10 newton-meters (50 newtons multiplied by 0.2 meters).

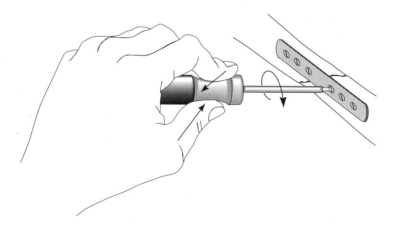

**Figure 1.3.** In removing a bone screw, a moment is created when the fingers apply a couple to the handle of the screwdriver.

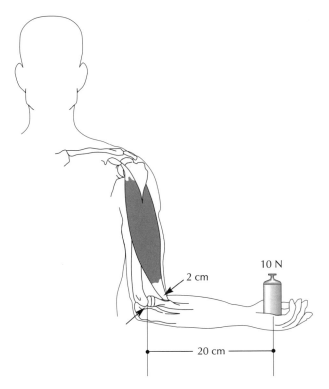

**Figure 1.4.** A 10-newton weight in the hand creates a 2-newton-meter moment about the elbow.

applied to the limb and by internal forces generated by muscle contractions. The magnitude of the moment created about the joint can be calculated as the product of the force and the perpendicular distance between the line of action of the force and the center of rotation of the joint. This distance is often called the moment arm of the force. Thus, the external force applied to the outstretched hand by the 10-newton weight in Figure 1.4 creates a moment of 2 newton-meters about the elbow (the 10-newton force multiplied by a moment arm of 0.2 meters). Note that the moment arm of the biceps muscle about the elbow is an order of magnitude smaller (0.02 meters) than the moment arm of the 10-newton weight (0.2 meters), so the muscle must generate 10 times the force to create the same magnitude moment about the elbow as was created by the 10-newton weight.

## STATIC EQUILIBRIUM

Equipped with the concepts of force and moment, we can begin to investigate important questions concerning the mechanics of the musculoskeletal system. Questions such as how much muscle force the patient must provide to maintain the arm in an outstretched position, how much force is applied to the head of the femur and across the knee joint when the patient rises from a chair, and how much force is applied across the knee joint during a maximal isometric contraction of the hamstring muscles, are important to consider in prescribing rehabilitation exercises after injury or surgery and in choosing implants and methods of implant fixation to support or replace portions of the musculoskeletal system.

How do we proceed to answer these questions? The easiest approach is to assume that, in each of these cases, there is no motion or virtually no change in motion. The two basic laws of mechanics that we used to define forces and moments still apply for all of the portions of the musculoskeletal system being considered. The expressions Force = Mass × Acceleration and Moment = (Mass moment of inertia)×(Angular acceleration) *define the force and moment necessary to create an acceleration.* But these expressions can also be interpreted for the special case where there is no acceleration. For the case of no acceleration, the two laws simplify to

$$\sum \text{Forces} = 0 \tag{1.3}$$

$$\sum \text{Moments} = 0 \tag{1.4}$$

where the symbol $\sum$ means that the net force (the sum of all the forces) or the net moment (the sum of all the moments) acting on the object or the part of the object that is not accelerating must be zero.

For example, a person standing stationary on a bathroom scale is not experiencing any acceleration (Fig. 1.5). The person's 71-kilogram mass is pushing down on the scale with a gravity force of 700 newtons. To maintain the person's stationary position, the ground—or in this case the bathroom scale—must be pushing up on the person's body with an equal and oppositely directed 700-newton force. The two forces on the person (the gravity force and the ground reaction force) exactly counteract one another, so that the net force is zero.

The formal statement of this common but special case of Newton's law (Equation 1.1) is that *if the acceleration of an object is zero, the net force and the net moment acting on the object are zero. The object is said to be in a state of equilibrium.* So if there is no acceleration, the forces and the moments on the object will add to zero.

When we examine an object to determine the forces or moments acting on that object, *the object is called a free body.* A free body can be made from any object or portion of an object by defining the object or the portion of the object as being within an imaginary boundary. For the example of the person standing on the bathroom scale (Fig. 1.5), the free body is the entire person, so that the boundary of the free body passes around the entire person. No portion of the person is outside the boundary, and no other object (such as the scale) is within the boundary.

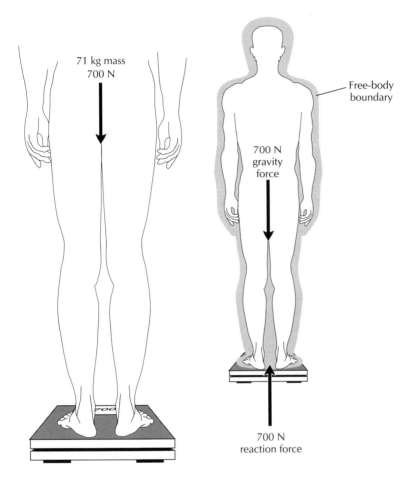

**Figure 1.5.** Under the influence of gravity, the mass of the person creates a downward force of 700 newtons. Equilibrium requires that the bathroom scale push up on the person's body with an equal and opposite force of 700 newtons.

The free body must also contain all the forces and moments acting across the boundary of the free body. Note that gravity forces always act across the free-body boundary. For the person on the bathroom scale, only two forces act across the free-body boundary: the gravity force and the reaction force of the scale pushing up on the person's feet. If the magnitude of the reaction force were unknown, as it was before the person stepped on the scale, we could apply the law of mechanics for equilibrium (net force = 0 when acceleration = 0). For equilibrium, the magnitude of reaction force required to be added to the 700-newton gravity force is a force of 700 newtons pushing up on the body in the opposite direction (a negatively directed force of 700 newtons, as shown in Fig. 1.5).

## PROBLEMS SOLVED ASSUMING STATIC EQUILIBRIUM

### Choosing an Appropriate Free Body

Returning to the first of our four questions, that of what the muscle force would be across the shoulder to maintain the arm in an outstretched position, we must first choose the free body to be considered. We take the arm as the free body and choose a boundary around the entire arm, passing through the shoulder joint between the glenoid and the head of the humerus and cutting across the muscles, ligaments, and capsular structures of the shoulder joint.

Next we must account for all the forces acting across the free-body boundary (Fig. 1.6). These include the gravity force caused by the mass of the arm, the joint reaction force of the glenoid pushing on the humeral head, and the forces of the muscles and other soft-tissue structures that cross the boundary and pull on the arm. Some judgment is required in selecting which muscle and soft-tissue forces to include across the boundary. A knowledge of anatomy is necessary to decide which muscles would exert force to abduct the arm and to decide if there could be tension in any of the soft-tissue structures (ligaments and capsule) for the position of the arm being considered. For our example, we will consider the deltoid muscle to be the only muscle actively resisting the moment created by the gravity force.

Remember that internal forces that do not cross the free-body boundary are not considered and do not influence the equilibrium of the arm. For example,

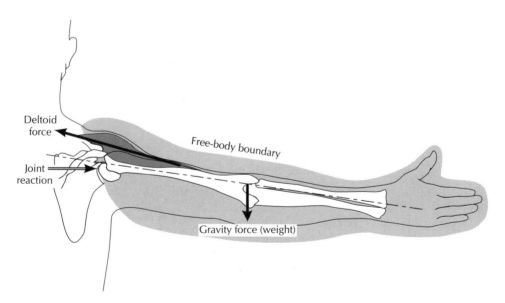

**Figure 1.6.** A free-body diagram of the arm including the three forces that cross the boundary of the free body (the gravity force caused by the mass of the arm, the joint reaction force on the humerus from the glenoid, and the force of the deltoid muscle contraction).

the forces at the elbow joint do not cross the boundary and therefore do not influence the equilibrium of the arm. As an extreme example, the elbow could be fused, eliminating the joint reaction forces between the distal humerus and the radius and ulna. The forces at the shoulder required to maintain the arm in equilibrium would not change from the case in which the elbow is not fused.

As another example of choosing an appropriate free body, consider our second question, concerning the joint reaction force at the hip joint when a person rises from a chair. What segment of the person should we choose as the free body to determine the forces on the head of the left femur? Certainly, the free-body boundary must pass through the hip joint just over the head of the femur if the force across the hip joint is to be included in the analysis.

Two possible free bodies could be chosen (Fig. 1.7). The free body could be constructed to include the superincumbent body and contralateral limb (the torso, the upper extremities, the head, and the right leg). The second choice would be to construct the free body to include only the lower limb. We choose the latter, because there are fewer potential forces acting across the boundary.

The forces that cross the free-body boundary of the lower limb are the gravity force caused by the mass of the lower limb, the reaction force of the ground pushing upward on the foot, the force of the acetabulum pushing on the head of the femur, and the force of the gluteus muscle pulling on the proximal femur to extend the leg. Note again that forces internal to the free-body boundary are not included. For example, forces acting about the knee joint, such as the tension of the short head of the quadriceps muscle tending to extend the knee, the joint contact force between the femur and the tibia, and the force in the patellar ligament, need not be considered since they do not influence the state of equilibrium of the lower-limb free body that we have chosen. As another extreme example, we can imagine the knee joint to be fused in the position shown in Figure 1.7. There would be no effect on any of the forces we have described acting on the free body of the limb.

## Making Assumptions about Forces

**Friction** In assigning forces across the free-body boundary, all known properties of the force must be maintained. In the case of joint contact forces, the property of the joint surface related to slipperiness imposes strict limitations on the direction of the force. When the two surfaces of a total knee joint replacement are compressed against one another and then forced to slide relative to one another, the force across the surface may be thought of as having two components: a normal component acting perpendicular to the joint surface and a tangential component acting parallel to the surface (Fig. 1.8). Another way of describing this situation is to say that the force is acting in such a direction that it is tilted relative to the surface.

*The ratio of the tangential component to the normal component is called the coefficient of friction.* Viewed in terms of the direction of the contact force, *the coefficient of friction is the tangent of the angle at which the force*

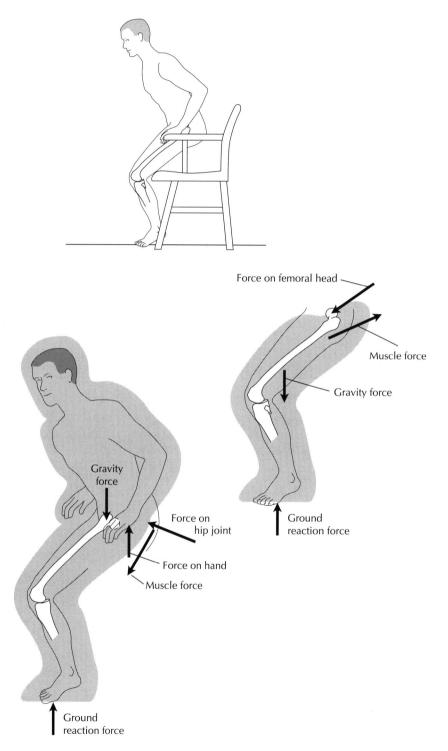

**Figure 1.7.** Two possible free bodies for examining the forces across the left hip joint.

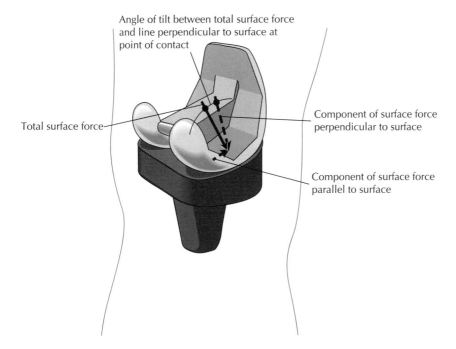

Angle of tilt between total surface force
and line perpendicular to surface at
point of contact

Total surface force

Component of surface force
perpendicular to surface

Component of surface force
parallel to surface

**Figure 1.8.** The force acting across a surface between two bodies has a component perpendicular to the surface and a component parallel to the surface. The coefficient of friction can be thought of either as the ratio of the amplitude of the parallel component to the perpendicular component or as the tangent of the angle of tilt of the surface force.

*is tilted* (Fig. 1.8). For example, two finely polished surfaces of cobalt alloy, such as those that formed the articulating surfaces of the original McKee-Farrar hip replacement, have a coefficient of friction of 0.15, corresponding to a maximum tilt angle of the contact force of 8.5 degrees. For the more contemporary combination of polished cobalt alloy articulating against ultra-high-molecular-weight polyethylene, the coefficient is 0.05, corresponding to a tilt angle of less than 3 degrees for the contact force. Finally, for the natural joint in which cartilage articulates against cartilage, the coefficient is 0.002, leading to a maximum possible tilt angle of only a tenth of a degree.

For normal joints, therefore, it is reasonable to assume that the joint contact force is perpendicular to the joint surface. For curved surfaces, a line of action that is perpendicular to the surface also passes through the center of curvature of the surface. Most of the common joints in the body consist of curved surfaces, so that the contact force across the joint will be perpendicular to the joint surface and will pass through the center of curvature of the joint.

**Line of Action of Muscle and Ligament Forces** Whenever we construct a free body of a limb or other body segment, we must include those forces caused by muscle or ligament acting across the free-body boundary. Muscle forces are usually considered to act along the direction of a line passing through the center of the muscle. The muscle center is assumed to be the centroid (the center of area) of the muscle cross-section. Thus, in the free body of the left leg shown in Figure 1.7, the muscle force contributed by the gluteus muscle is represented as a force acting across the boundary along a line that is parallel to the long axis of the muscle and that passes through the centroid of the cross-section of the muscle belly.

Ligament forces can usually be considered to act along the anatomical axis of the tensed ligament. For simple ligament structures, such as the patellar ligament connecting the tibia and the patella, this line of action is assumed to be parallel to the direction along which the ligament fibers are aligned and to pass through the center of the cross-section of the ligament. For more complex ligament structures, such as the anterior cruciate ligament of the knee, with twisted fiber bundles or fiber bundles in more than one common direction, average directions are often assumed. If such an approach is impractical, the ligament force may be broken into components along the variously directed bundles.

### Solving the Problem by Considering Force Components in Horizontal and Vertical Directions

Now let's return to the first of our three static equilibrium questions, illustrated in Figure 1.6. We want to determine the muscle force across the shoulder and the compressive joint reaction force on the head of the humerus. To find these two quantities, we apply the two statements of equilibrium:

1. With no acceleration (no change in velocity), all forces must sum to zero (the net force on the free body is zero).
2. With no angular acceleration (no change in angular velocity), all moments must sum to zero (the net moment on the free body is zero).

The conventional way to add and subtract forces is to resolve them into horizontal and vertical components. The horizontal and vertical components can then be dealt with separately, since only the horizontal components of the force will affect horizontal acceleration of the free body, and only the vertical components of the force will affect vertical acceleration. In fact, any two directions can be considered in such an approach, as long as they are perpendicular to one another. In our question concerning the shoulder, for example, the forces can just as easily be resolved into components perpendicular and parallel to the long axis of the arm.

To resolve a force into two perpendicular components, consider the force as forming the diagonal of a rectangle (Fig. 1.9). The sides of the rectangle will represent the magnitudes and directions of the two components. For the free body of the shoulder, the gravity force created by the weight of the arm has a vertical component of 50 newtons. The horizontal component of the gravity force is zero, since by definition gravity forces are vertically directed toward the center of the earth.

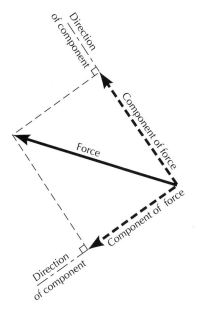

**Figure 1.9.** A force can be broken into components by considering the force to be the diagonal of a rectangle.

While we know from anatomy the orientation of the muscle force across the shoulder joint (Fig. 1.10A), we do not know the magnitude of the muscle force. However, the orientation does allow us to determine the relative magnitudes of the vertical and horizontal components. With the muscle force oriented at 15 degrees from the horizontal direction, the vertical ($F_V$) and horizontal ($F_H$) components are related as

$$F_V = F_H \times \tan(15°) = F_H \times 0.27$$

We do not know the direction or the magnitude of the joint contact force, so the horizontal ($J_H$) and vertical ($J_V$) components are completely unknown.

We can now sum the forces in the vertical direction and use the condition of equilibrium (Equation 1.3) to set the sum equal to zero:

$$F_V - J_V - 50\,\text{N} = 0$$

Note that we have adopted a convention in which forces acting in the superior vertical direction are positive quantities, while forces acting in the inferior vertical direction are negative quantities. Substituting for the vertical component of the muscle force, the equation for the vertical force components becomes

$$(F_H \times 0.27) - J_V - 50\,\text{N} = 0$$

Similarly, we can use the equilibrium condition (Equation 1.3) to sum the forces in the horizontal direction and set the sum equal to zero:

$$F_H - J_H = 0$$

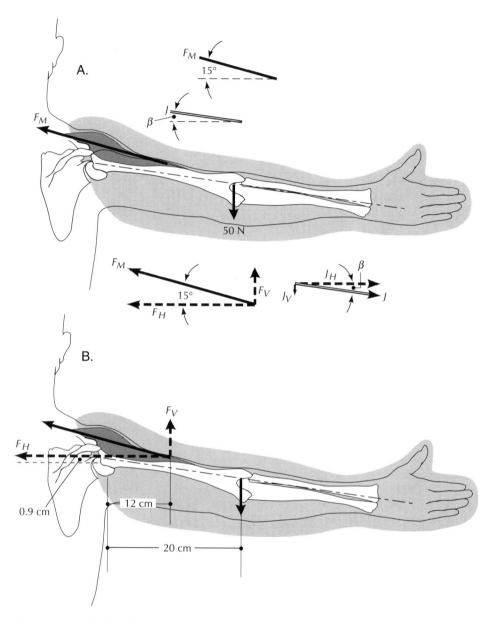

**Figure 1.10.** The free body of the arm (Fig. 1.6) showing the vertical and horizontal components of the three forces acting across the free-body boundary. The moment arms about the joint contact point for the gravity force and the horizontal and vertical muscle force components are also shown.

Note that our convention for the horizontal forces is that positive quantities represent those forces acting toward the body, in a proximal horizontal direction, and negative quantities represent those forces acting away from the body, in a distal horizontal direction.

Finally, we can use the law of mechanics (Equation 1.4), which states that the sum of the moments acting on a free body in equilibrium is zero, to write a third equation. To develop this equation, we need to choose a point on the free body about which to sum the moments. The clever choice is a point about which one of the unknown forces creates no moment, which would eliminate the unknown force from the moment equation. A good choice in this particular problem is the center of curvature of the joint contact surface, since the joint contact force that must pass through this point produces no moment about this point.

The moment equation about the joint center therefore includes only the moment $(M_G)$ created by the gravity force (50 newtons), the moment produced by the vertical component $(F_V)$ of the muscle force, and the moment produced by the horizontal component $(F_H)$ of the muscle force:

$$M_G - M_{F_V} + M_{F_H} = 0$$

Note that we have also adopted a sign convention for the moments. Moments that would tend to move the arm in adduction are positive quantities, and moments that would tend to move the arm in abduction are negative quantities.

We can determine the moment arms of the gravity force and the two components of the muscle force from the anatomy of the arm in the extended position (Fig. 1.10B). The moment arm of the gravity force is 0.2 meters. The moment arms of the vertical and horizontal components of the muscle force are 0.12 and 0.009 meters, respectively. Substituting for the magnitudes of the moments in terms of the force multiplied by the moment arm, the moment equation becomes

$$(50 \text{ N} \times 0.2 \text{ m}) - (F_V \times 0.12 \text{ m}) + (F_H \times 0.009 \text{ m}) = 0$$

We can substitute for the vertical component of the muscle force $(F_V)$ in terms of the horizontal component $(F_H)$ using the previous relationship obtained by trigonometry:

$$F_V = F_H \times 0.27$$

The moment equation then becomes

$$(50 \text{ N} \times 0.2 \text{ m}) - (F_H \times 0.27 \times 0.12 \text{ m}) + (F_H \times 0.009 \text{ m}) = 0$$

$$(50 \text{ N} \times 0.2 \text{ m}) - (F_H \times 0.041 \text{ m}) = 0$$

We now have three equations (the sum of the forces in the vertical direction, the sum of the forces in the horizontal direction, and the sum of the moments about the joint center) containing three unknown quantities (the horizontal component of the muscle force and the horizontal and vertical components of the joint reaction force). We can now find the solution in a straightforward manner by solving the moment equation for the horizontal muscle force component ($F_H$):

$$F_H = 244 \text{ N}$$

This value can then be substituted into the second equation, for the sum of the forces in the horizontal direction, to solve for the horizontal joint contact force component ($J_H$). Because there are only two force components in the horizontal direction, the force component $J_H$ will have the same magnitude as the horizontal muscle force component:

$$J_H = 244 \text{ N}$$

Similarly, $F_H$ can be substituted into the first equation, for the sum of the forces in the vertical direction, to solve for $J_V$:

$$J_V = 16 \text{ N}$$

The components can then be used to calculate the magnitude of the muscle force, as well as the direction and magnitude of the joint reaction force:

$$F_M = F_H \times \frac{1}{\cos(15°)} = 253 \text{ N}$$

$$\beta = \tan^{-1}\left(\frac{J_V}{J_H}\right) = 3.75°$$

$$J = J_V \times \frac{1}{\sin(3.75°)} = 245 \text{ N}$$

Note that the angle $\beta$, as shown in Figure 1.10, is measured relative to the horizontal axis. Note also that the magnitudes of the muscle force and the joint reaction force are quite large, about five times the gravity force.

### Solving the Problem by Considering Force Components in Directions Perpendicular and Parallel to the Axis of the Bone

A second way to solve the same problem is to resolve the forces applied across the free-body boundary of the arm into components perpendicular and parallel to the long axis of the arm. This process is made simpler by understanding that, as far as the conditions of equilibrium are concerned, the effect of a force is the same no matter where along the line of action the force is assumed to be applied. Consider, for example, the gravity force (whose line of action passes through the center of gravity of the arm in a vertical direction) to be applied at a point on the long axis of the humerus (Fig. 1.11). Also, consider the muscle force (whose line of action passes along the central axis of the muscle) to be applied at a point where its line of action crosses the long axis of the humerus.

The reason for these considerations becomes more obvious when we re-solve these forces into components perpendicular and parallel to the axis of the humerus. Note that now the component of the gravity force parallel to the humeral axis, the component of the muscle force parallel to the axis, and both components of the joint reaction force have their lines of action passing through the point of contact between the glenoid and the humerus on the joint contact surface.

We can now solve the problem in much the same way as before, using the conditions of equilibrium (Equations 1.3 and 1.4) to sum the components of force perpendicular to the humeral axis to zero, the components of force paral-lel to the humeral axis to zero, and the moments about the joint contact point to zero. The equation resulting from the last equilibrium condition is simpli-fied, since the only two components creating a moment (that is, having a finite moment arm) about the joint contact point are the components of the gravity force and the muscle force perpendicular to the humeral axis.

The measured moment arm of the gravity force component $(G_\perp)$ is 0.2 meters divided by the cosine of 8 degrees (Fig. 1.10), and the moment arm of the muscle force component $(F_\perp)$ is 0.32 meters (Fig. 1.11). Using the same

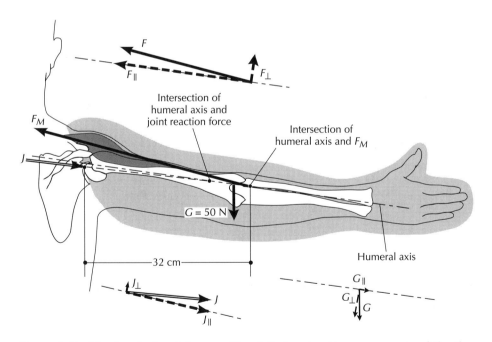

**Figure 1.11.** The free body of the arm (Fig. 1.6) showing the components of the three forces perpendicular and parallel to the axis of the humerus.

sign convention for positive and negative moments as was used in our first solution of this problem, the equilibrium equation (Equation 1.4) for the sum of the moments about the joint contact point becomes

$$\left(G_\perp \times \frac{0.2\ \text{m}}{\cos(8°)}\right) - (F_\perp \times 0.32\ \text{m}) = 0$$

The orientation of the gravity force relative to the arm is known, so that the perpendicular component can be calculated:

$$G_\perp = 50\ \text{N} \times \cos(8°)$$

With this value for $G_\perp$ substituted into the equilibrium moment equation, $F_\perp$ can be calculated:

$$50\ \text{N} \times \cos(8°) \times \frac{0.2\ \text{m}}{\cos(8°)} - (F_\perp \times 0.32\ \text{m}) = 0$$

$$F_\perp = 50\ \text{N} \times \left(\frac{0.2\ \text{m}}{0.32\ \text{m}}\right) = 31.2\ \text{N}$$

As in our first solution to this problem, we know the orientation of the muscle force. Therefore, we know the relative magnitudes of the perpendicular $(F_\perp)$ and parallel $(F_\parallel)$ components of the muscle force, giving us the ability to solve for the other unknown quantities, the components of the joint reaction force, using the two conditions for force equilibrium. The equilibrium condition for the forces acting perpendicular to the humeral axis is

$$F_\perp + J_\perp - G_\perp = 0$$

Substituting the values already calculated for the first two components results in

$$J_\perp = 18.3\ \text{N}$$

The equilibrium condition for the forces acting parallel to the humeral axis is

$$F_\parallel - J_\parallel - G_\parallel = 0$$

Again, because we know the orientation of the gravity and muscle forces relative to the arm, we can calculate $G_\parallel$ and $F_\parallel$:

$$G_\parallel = G_\perp \times \tan(8°) = 7.0\ \text{N}$$

$$F_\parallel = F_\perp \times \frac{1}{\tan(7°)} = 254.1\ \text{N}$$

Substituting these values into the equilibrium equation, we can calculate $J_\parallel$:

$$J_\parallel = 247.1 \text{ N}$$

All the components of the forces are now known, so we can determine the magnitude of the muscle force and the direction and magnitude of the joint reaction force in the same fashion as we did in our first solution to the problem:

$$F_M = F_\perp \times \frac{1}{\sin(7°)} = 256 \text{ N}$$

$$\alpha = \tan^{-1}\left(\frac{J_\perp}{J_\parallel}\right) = 4.24°$$

$$J = J_\parallel \times \frac{1}{\cos(4.24°)} = 248 \text{ N}$$

Note that the answers for the magnitudes of the muscle and joint reaction forces are in close agreement with the values calculated in our previous solution, in which we considered components in the vertical and horizontal directions. Note also that the angle $\alpha$ in this solution is not the same as the angle $\beta$ in the previous solution. In the first solution, $\beta$ was 3.75 degrees as measured from the horizontal axis. In this solution, $\alpha$ is 4.24 degrees as measured from the axis of the humerus. But the humerus itself is oriented at 8 degrees from the horizontal. The orientation from the horizontal is therefore 3.76 degrees (8 degrees − 4.24 degrees), in close agreement with the first solution.

### Solving the Problem by Adding Forces Graphically

A third method involves a graphical technique that can be used to solve equilibrium problems in the musculoskeletal system. This technique can be used whenever only three forces are acting on the free body. This type of problem is quite common, and many complex problems involving more than three forces can often be accurately approximated as a simple three-force problem. The most common three-force problems involve a functional force (such as gravity or an applied force), a muscle force (required to overcome the rotational tendency of the joint created by the functional force), and a reaction force across the joint caused by the combined action of the other two forces.

To find the muscle force and the joint reaction at the shoulder, we again apply the two statements of equilibrium. Of the three forces acting on the free body (Fig. 1.12A), we usually know the magnitude and orientation of the functional force. If the functional force is due to gravity, the magnitude will be equal to the weight and the direction will be vertical. From anatomy, we can also assume the orientation of the muscle force. Finally, we know that

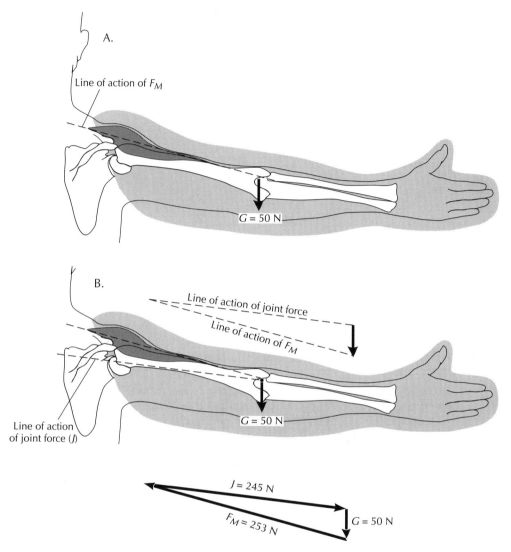

A.

Line of action of $F_M$

$G = 50$ N

B.

Line of action of joint force

Line of action of $F_M$

$G = 50$ N

Line of action
of joint force ($J$)

$J = 245$ N

$F_M = 253$ N

$G = 50$ N

**Figure 1.12.** Graphical construction of a force triangle to solve for the magnitude of the deltoid muscle force and the joint reaction force at the shoulder.

the joint reaction force passes through the center of curvature of the two joint surfaces, though we do not know its magnitude or orientation.

In applying the statement of equilibrium of the moments applied to the free body, note that if we extend the lines of action of the functional force and the muscle force, they will pass through a common point. The moment produced by the functional force about the intersection point of the two lines of action must be zero, because the moment arm of the functional force about this point is zero. The moment produced by the muscle force about this point is also zero, for the same reason. Since moment equilibrium requires that the sum of the moments of all forces acting on the free body be zero about any point, we come to an interesting deduction. Because the moments must sum to zero about this point, then the moment produced by the joint reaction force about this point must also be zero. Physically, the joint reaction force can be oriented so as to create no moment only if the line of action of the reaction force also passes through the common intersection point. We thus have the geometric corollary that *if the free body is in equilibrium under the influence of three forces, the lines of action of the three forces must be concurrent.*

This corollary allows us to determine the orientation of the joint reaction force simply by drawing a line from the center of the joint to the intersecting point of the lines of action of the other two forces. Thus, the principle of moment equilibrium tells us the orientation of the joint reaction force. Another geometric corollary can be deduced from the equilibrium condition, which states that the sum of the forces must equal zero. This statement is equivalent to having the arrows that represent the directions and magnitudes of the three forces form the sides of a triangle. If the net force is zero (that is, if a condition of equilibrium exists), the three forces will form a closed triangle, with the head of the third force arrow meeting the tail of the first arrow.

To find the magnitude of the muscle force and the magnitude of the joint reaction force, we start by scaling the gravity force (functional force) arrow so that the length of the arrow equals the known magnitude. At the head of this arrow, we construct a line parallel to the known orientation of the line of action of the muscle force (Fig. 1.12$A$). We do not know the magnitude of the muscle force, so we do not know how long to make the arrow along this line. We can determine the orientation (line of action) of the joint reaction force ($J$) since the force must pass through both the joint contact point and the intersection of the line of action of the muscle force ($F_M$) and the line of action of the gravity force ($G$). We also know that the line of action of the joint reaction force must pass through the origin of the gravity force arrow (Fig. 1.12$B$), since we know that the joint reaction force must form the third side of the triangle.

Now all three sides of the triangle are complete (Fig. 1.12$B$). Using our scale that relates the magnitude of the gravity force to the length of the arrow representing the gravity force, we can measure the lengths of the arrows for the muscle and joint reaction forces and determine their magnitudes.

## Another Example of Solving a Problem by Considering Force Components in Horizontal and Vertical Directions

Let us now return to the second question we raised, concerning the forces across the hip joint in a patient rising from a chair (Fig. 1.13). We now choose a free body of one lower limb to determine the force on the left hip joint. The free-body boundary passes through the left hip joint between the femur and the acetabulum. The forces acting across the boundary are the reaction force ($R$) of the ground pushing up on the foot, the force of the gluteus muscle ($F_M$) pulling on the femur to extend the hip joint, and the joint reaction force ($J$) of the acetabulum pushing down on the femoral head.

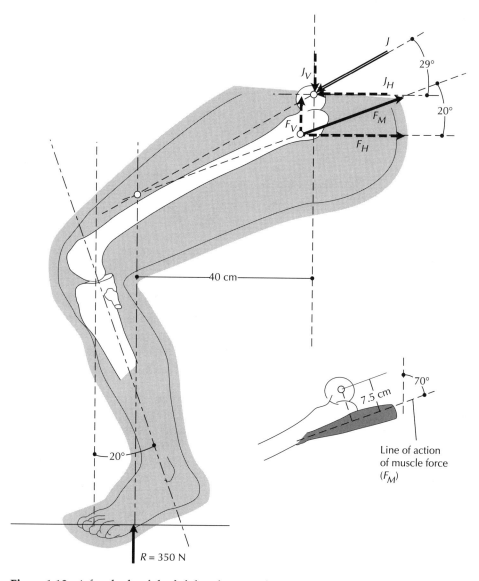

**Figure 1.13.** A free body of the left leg showing the vertical and horizontal components of the three forces crossing the free-body boundary.

To find the joint reaction force, we will begin by summing the horizontal components of the forces and setting the sum equal to zero, as dictated by equilibrium. The ground reaction force acts along a vertical direction and therefore has no horizontal component. The unknown muscle and joint reaction forces both have horizontal components, so that the equilibrium equation (Equation 1.3) becomes

$$F_H - J_H = 0$$

Next we will sum the vertical components and set the sum equal to zero for equilibrium. All three forces acting across the free-body boundary have vertical components. The vertical component of the ground reaction force $(R)$ is the force itself, since it acts in a vertical direction. The magnitude of this force is 350 newtons, assuming a body weight of 800 newtons distributed equally on both feet, with a portion (100 newtons) of body weight supported by the patient using the arm rests of the chair (Fig. 1.7). The vertical components of the other two forces are unknown, so the equilibrium equation (Equation 1.3) becomes

$$350 \text{ N} + F_V - J_V = 0$$

By observing the anatomy around the hip joint, we can obtain the orientation of the gluteus muscle. The muscle acts along a direction oriented at 70 degrees from the vertical for the position of the leg shown in Figure 1.13. Because the orientation is known, the relation between the relative magnitudes of the vertical and horizontal components of the muscle force can be obtained:

$$F_V = F_H \times \frac{1}{\tan(70°)} = F_H \times 0.36$$

Substituting this expression into the equilibrium equation for the vertical force components yields

$$350 \text{ N} + (F_H \times 0.36) - J_V = 0$$

We can now use the other equilibrium condition to develop an equation for the sum of the moments on the lower limb about the joint center. This sum must equal zero, since although the limb is moving slowly, we are assuming the limb to be in equilibrium. By choosing the joint center as the point about which to sum the moments, we can eliminate one of the unknown forces from the equation, namely, the joint reaction force. This is possible because the joint reaction force and hence its components act in directions that pass through the joint center. They have no moment arm about this point and therefore cannot generate a moment.

The only forces acting on the limb that generate moments about the joint center are the ground reaction force and the muscle force. In the answer to our first question, concerning the forces at the shoulder, we constructed the moment equilibrium equation by considering the separate moments created by the vertical and horizontal components of the muscle force acting on the arm. In the present solution, let's consider the moment created by the muscle force $(F_M)$ itself.

The moment arms for the ground reaction force and the muscle force can be measured by considering the geometry of the leg in the position being studied

(Fig. 1.13). The magnitudes of the moments must sum to zero for equilibrium (Equation 1.4), so

$$(F_M \times 0.075 \text{ m}) - (R \times 0.4 \text{ m}) = 0$$

Because we know the orientation of the muscle force, we can develop a relation between the muscle force and one of its components:

$$F_M = F_H \times \frac{1}{\sin(70°)} = F_H \times 1.064$$

Substituting this expression into the moment equation, along with the known magnitude of the ground reaction force (350 newtons), gives an expression that can be solved for the horizontal component of the muscle force:

$$(F_H \times 1.064 \times 0.075 \text{ m}) - (350 \text{ N} \times 0.4 \text{ m}) = 0$$

$$F_H = 1754 \text{ N}$$

We can now substitute this value into the equilibrium equations for the forces in the horizontal and vertical directions to find the two components of the joint reaction force:

$$J_H = 1754 \text{ N}$$

$$J_V = 981 \text{ N}$$

We now have the necessary information to solve for the magnitude of the force generated by the gluteus muscle, and for the orientation and magnitude of the joint reaction force on the femoral head:

$$F_M = F_H \times \frac{1}{\sin(70°)} = 1867 \text{ N}$$

$$\gamma = \tan^{-1}\left(\frac{J_V}{J_H}\right) = 29°$$

$$J = J_V \times \frac{1}{\sin(29°)} = 2023 \text{ N}$$

Note that the magnitudes of the force in the gluteus muscle and of the joint reaction force on the femur are quite high, about 2 1/3 and 2 1/2 times body weight, respectively. Of course, the magnitudes of these two forces would be even higher if the patient's weight were not partly supported on the arms of the chair. Remember, this assumption decreased the total ground reaction force on both feet from 800 newtons to 700 newtons.

Note also the direction of the joint reaction force on the femur. In our two-dimensional solution to the problem, the forces on the free body were all assumed to act in the same sagittal plane, and the angle ($\gamma$) of the line of action of the joint reaction force was calculated to be 29 degrees as measured up from the horizontal direction (Fig. 1.13), with the joint reaction force pushing down on the head of the femur. We arrived at this solution based on the assumption that the ground reaction force, the muscle force, and the joint reaction force are all coplanar.

This assumption made our problem easy to solve, but the anatomy of the hip joint suggests that in the real, three-dimensional case, the directions of the forces would probably not lie in a sagittal plane. For example, three-dimensional studies of the forces at the hip joint during the act of rising from a chair (1) have found the joint reaction force to be pointed in a direction generally parallel with the femur, in reasonable agreement with our solution. But the joint reaction force was also shown to have a significant component out of the sagittal plane in the lateral direction, an understandable result considering the anatomy of the muscles acting at the hip joint during the activity of rising from a chair.

### Another Example of Solving a Problem by Considering Force Components in Directions Perpendicular and Parallel to the Axis of the Bone

Now consider our third question, concerning the forces about the knee joint during the act of rising from a chair. We choose as our free body the lower leg (Fig. 1.14). The free-body boundary passes through the knee joint between the femoral and tibial joint surfaces, and through the patellar ligament. The forces that cross this boundary are the reaction force ($R$) of the ground pushing up on the foot, the force of the patellar ligament ($P$) created by the pull of the quadriceps muscle, and the joint reaction force ($J$) of the femur pushing down on the tibia.

To solve this problem, we will use the two equilibrium conditions. First, we will solve for the components of the unknown forces perpendicular and parallel to the long axis of the tibia by setting both the sum of the perpendicular force components to zero and the sum of the parallel force components to zero, as dictated by equilibrium conditions. Our second equilibrium condition will allow us to set the sum of the moments acting on the lower leg about a point equal to zero. As in our earlier examples, the point about which we choose to sum moments is the joint center, since the components of the joint reaction force and the patellar ligament force that are parallel to the tibial axis generate no moment about the joint center. Remember that we have extended the line of action of the patellar ligament force so that its point of application is on the tibial axis, rather than on the surface of the tibia. Therefore, the moment of its component parallel to the tibial axis is indeed zero, since it, too, passes through the joint center.

We begin our solution by adding together the force components parallel to the tibial axis and setting the sum equal to zero. Both the orientation and

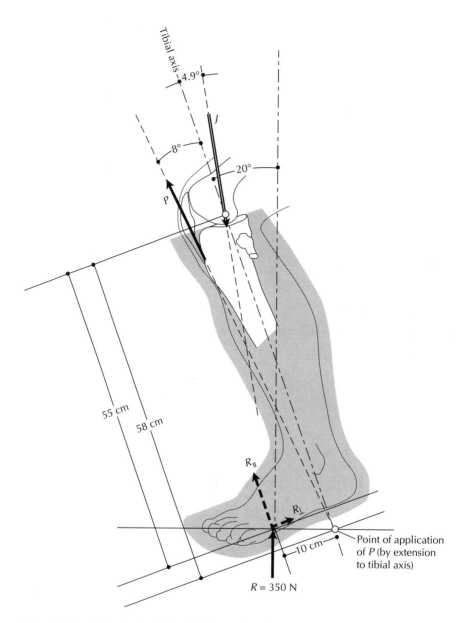

**Figure 1.14.** A free body of the left lower leg showing the force components perpendicular and parallel to the tibia for the three forces crossing the free-body boundary. All dimensions are as measured on a radiograph.

magnitude of the ground reaction force are known quantities. For the position of the lower leg in Figure 1.14, the orientation of the ground reaction force ($R$) relative to the tibial axis is 20 degrees. The magnitude of $R$ is 350 newtons, the same as was used in our earlier example concerning the hip joint. The component of the ground reaction force parallel to the tibial axis is

$$R_\parallel = R \times \cos(20°) = 329 \text{ N}$$

The patellar ligament force as transposed along its line of action to the tibial axis also has a component parallel to the tibial axis. We do not know the magnitude of the force (or of its components), but because the patellar ligament is a simple structure with its fiber bundles aligned along the long axis of the ligament, we can portray the force as having a line of action along the central axis of the ligament. The orientation of the patellar ligament force can be obtained by observing the anatomy of the leg. For the position shown in Figure 1.14, the ligament force is oriented at 8 degrees to the tibial axis. The relative magnitudes of the components of $P$ are therefore

$$P_\parallel = P_\perp \times \frac{1}{\tan(8°)} = P_\perp \times 7.1$$

Finally, the joint reaction force also has a component parallel to the tibial axis, though its magnitude is also unknown. The equilibrium condition (Equation 1.3) requiring that the components of force parallel to the tibial axis equal zero becomes

$$-R_\parallel - P_\parallel + J_\parallel = 0$$

Substituting our known values for $R_\parallel$ and $P_\parallel$, the equilibrium equation becomes

$$-329 \text{ N} - (P_\perp \times 7.1) + J_\parallel = 0$$

The second equilibrium condition, that the forces perpendicular to the tibial axis must also equal zero, leads to the relation

$$R_\perp - P_\perp - J_\perp = 0$$

Again, the orientation and magnitude of the ground reaction force are known, so $R_\perp$ becomes

$$R_\perp = R \times \sin(20°) = 120 \text{ N}$$

This value can be substituted into the equilibrium expression:

$$120 \text{ N} - P_\perp - J_\perp = 0$$

For our other equilibrium equation, we sum the moments acting on the lower leg about the joint center and set the sum equal to zero. The moment arms of the force components that generate moments about this point can be physically measured or scaled from a photograph (the values are shown in Fig. 1.14). The equation for moment equilibrium (Equation 1.4) is

$$-(R_\| \times 0.10 \text{ m}) + (R_\perp \times 0.58 \text{ m}) - (P_\perp \times 0.58 \text{ m}) = 0$$

Substituting the known values for the magnitudes of the components of $R$ perpendicular and parallel to the tibial axis, and solving for $P_\perp$ results in

$$-(329 \text{ N} \times 0.10 \text{ m}) + (120 \text{ N} \times 0.55 \text{ m}) - (P_\perp \times 0.58 \text{ m}) = 0$$

$$P_\perp = 57 \text{ N}$$

Substituting this value into the two equations that we developed for force equilibrium, we can solve for the two components of the joint reaction force:

$$J_\| = 734 \text{ N}$$

$$J_\perp = 63 \text{ N}$$

We can now solve the problem by calculating the magnitude of the patellar ligament force, and the orientation and magnitude of the joint reaction force:

$$P = P_\perp \times \frac{1}{\sin(8°)} = 410 \text{ N}$$

$$\theta = \tan^{-1}\left(\frac{J_\perp}{J_\|}\right) = 4.9°$$

$$J = J_\perp \times \frac{1}{\sin(4.9°)} = 737 \text{ N}$$

Note that the patellar ligament and joint reaction forces are large (about 1.2 and 2.1 times body weight, respectively), demonstrating that rising from a chair is indeed a strenuous activity, even when the patient uses the upper extremities to help support his or her weight.

### Another Example of Solving a Problem by Adding Forces Graphically

Our final static equilibrium question concerns the forces across the knee during a maximal isometric contraction of the hamstring muscles. This type of question is relevant when one is considering rehabilitation equipment such as Cybex and Lido machines. Such equipment allows the patient to conduct isometric or isokinetic exercises by generating a moment about a joint, such as the knee. In Figure 1.15 the patient is seen pushing against a pad at the ankle.

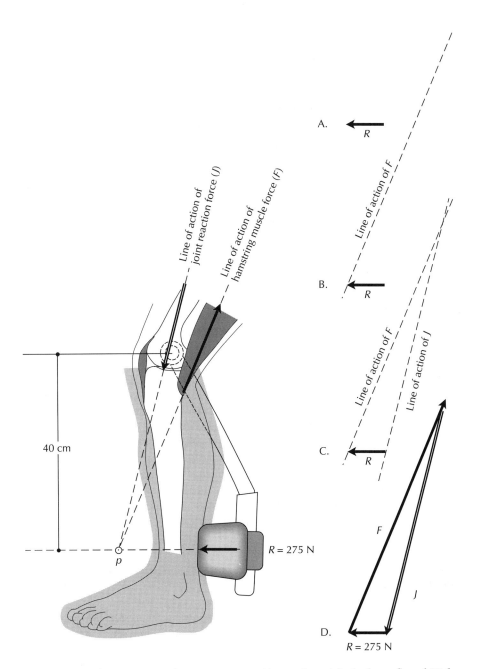

**Figure 1.15.** The patient performs an isometric exercise with the knee flexed 30 degrees. The machine registers a torque of 110 newton-meters. Since the moment arm of the machine is 0.4 meters (40 centimeters), the contact force (functional load, $R$) is 275 newtons. A force triangle is used to solve for the magnitude of the muscle force ($F$) and the joint reaction ($J$) from the known contact force ($R$) and directions of $F$ and $J$.

The pad is attached to an arm that rotates about an axle. The center of the axle is aligned with the knee joint center.

As the patient contracts the hamstring muscles, a force is produced against the pad, creating a moment about the knee. If the axle is prevented from rotating, the muscle contraction is isometric, and if the axle is allowed to rotate at a constant velocity, the muscle contraction is isokinetic. The question that we are concerned with deals with an isometric contraction of the hamstring muscles in an attempt by the patient to flex the knee joint against the resistance of the stationary pad. We want to know the force generated in the muscle and the joint reaction force generated at the knee.

An appropriate free body for this problem is the lower leg, with the boundary passing through the knee joint between the femur and the tibia, and through the patellar ligament. There are three forces that cross the boundary: the reaction force ($R$) of the pad pushing against the tibia, the force ($F$) of the hamstring muscles pulling on the tibia, and the reaction force ($J$) at the knee joint surface caused by the femur pushing on the tibia. Note that there is no force in the patellar ligament since there is no quadriceps muscle activity. Also, the weight of the lower leg is being ignored. The magnitude and orientation of the reaction force at the pad can be determined. The exercise equipment provides a measurement of the moment generated about the axle of the machine. Since the moment arm from the pad to the axle can be measured, the magnitude of the force can be calculated by dividing the measured moment by the measured moment arm. Because of the construction of the pad, the contact force is perpendicular to the arm of the machine.

In our problem, the patient generated a moment of 110 newton-meters during a maximal contraction of the hamstring muscles with the knee in 30 degrees of flexion (Fig. 1.15). The pad was placed 0.4 meters from the joint center of rotation. Therefore, the reaction force at the pad was 275 newtons (a moment of 110 newton-meters divided by a moment arm of 0.4 meters).

We will solve this problem using the graphical technique. Since we have a free body (the lower leg) in static equilibrium with only three applied forces, we can use our geometric corollary that all three forces must pass through a common point. Extending the lines of action of the reaction force at the pad and the muscle force on the tibia, we find that they intersect at point $p$. We assume the point of joint surface contact between the femur and tibia to be the midpoint of the joint surfaces. This is where the joint reaction force will be applied. We can construct the line of action of the joint reaction force, since it must pass through both point $p$ and the joint contact point.

We start by scaling the arrow representing the reaction force ($R$) so that by our scale the length of the arrow equals 275 newtons (Fig. 1.15A). At the head of this arrow we construct a line parallel to the known orientation of the line of action of the hamstring force ($F$) (Fig. 1.15B). We do not know how long to make the arrow along this line, because we do not know the magnitude of the muscle force. We do know the line of action of the joint reaction force ($J$), and we know that the arrow representing this force must pass through the origin of the reaction force arrow (Fig. 1.15C). Because the sum of these three forces must be zero for equilibrium, the joint reaction force must also complete the third side of a triangle. Using our scale that relates the length of the reaction force arrow to 275 newtons, we can determine the magnitudes of the muscle and joint reaction forces from the measured lengths of their arrows (Fig. 1.15D).

## Statically Indeterminate Problems

In all of the examples we just considered, it was possible to determine the unknown forces acting on the free body by employing the concept and equations of static equilibrium. A formal statement of the ability to solve these problems is that they are statically determinate. We were always able to develop as many equilibrium equations as there were unknown force quantities. There were always three unknown force magnitudes (the muscle force with its known line of action and two components of the joint reaction force with their unknown lines of action), and we were able to develop three equilibrium equations (by considering the sums of the forces in two perpendicular directions and the sum of the moments about a point).

Suppose, however, that we wanted to relax our assumption that only one muscle is active in resisting the functional force. For example, in our problem concerning the forces at the shoulder joint when the arm is held in an elevated position, we could more appropriately assume that both the deltoid and the supraspinatus muscles would be actively resisting the moment created by the gravity force. But the inclusion of additional unknown muscle forces leads to a situation in which the number of unknown quantities exceeds the number of equilibrium equations that we can develop to relate the quantities. While we can still find the relationships or ratios between the unknown quantities, we cannot find their absolute values. The problem becomes, therefore, statically indeterminate.

A method to solve statically indeterminate problems is to construct a scheme to divide the required resisting moment between the muscles. Such schemes to apportion the forces between the muscles are called optimization methods. As an example, in our problem to determine the force on the femoral head in rising from a chair, we assumed that only one muscle, the gluteus, was actively providing the necessary moment to extend the hip. A more detailed examination of the soft-tissue structures around the hip joint would reveal as many as 27 muscle and ligament structures that could potentially carry force that would create extension or flexion moments about the hip joint when the patient rises from a chair (1).

This more completely described, but more complicated, problem can be solved by applying an optimization method that assigns some rational way for relating the muscle forces. For example, the muscle forces could be apportioned on the basis of their cross-sectional area, or on the basis of minimizing the resulting joint reaction force or the resulting total force of all the muscles (2, 3). Once the proportionality among the muscle forces is assigned according to the optimization method, the equations of equilibrium are used to find the force magnitudes. None of the commonly used optimization strategies is apparently supported by any specific principles of physiology, but when several methods are applied to solve the same problem, the answers agree quite well (4).

The consideration of all muscles acting about a joint can make the solution of these problems more complicated in another way. Many of the muscles acting across one joint will also have an effect across an adjoining joint. Such muscles are called diarthroidal. For example, in our problem concerned with the force at the knee joint in rising from a chair, the ground reaction force that tends to flex the knee joint also tends to dorsiflex the ankle joint. Therefore, muscles that tend to plantar-flex the ankle must also be active. The gastrocnemius actively plantar-flexes the ankle joint but also tends to flex the knee.

In solving the problem of equilibrium at the knee joint, our calculated value for the gastrocnemius will have to be appropriate to maintain equilibrium at the ankle. Both problems, equilibrium at the knee joint and equilibrium at the ankle joint, must be solved separately, but the muscle forces obtained from the equilibrium solution to one problem must satisfy the equilibrium solution to the other problem. The choice of which muscles to include in the problem must be based on the muscles considered to be active. Electromyographic measurement is the most effective technique to determine whether a muscle is active, and such measurements are often included in experiments to determine the loading on joints during specific functions.

## DYNAMIC EQUILIBRIUM

Until now we have examined equilibrium situations in which there was neither acceleration nor angular acceleration of the body. However, human performance usually involves changes in velocity (that is, accelerations). Consider the foot during gait. In the stance phase of gait, the velocity of the foot is nearly zero, and its changes in velocity (its accelerations) are also nearly zero. But from toe-off to heel strike, the foot undergoes several changes in velocity, gaining velocity (accelerating) during the first half of the swing phase and then losing velocity (decelerating) during the second half of the swing phase, so that at heel strike its velocity is again zero.

Angular acceleration of the limbs also occurs during gait. During stance phase, the thigh is clearly seen rotating in the clockwise direction (Fig. 1.16). This is in contrast to the counterclockwise rotation of the thigh during swing phase. The change in angular velocity between these two motions means that the thigh is undergoing angular acceleration.

The stance phase of normal gait requires angular accelerations that are significantly less than those that occur during the swing phase. Indeed, many researchers have found that in determining the muscle and joint reaction forces in stance phase, the accelerations can be ignored. This results in a static equilibrium problem whose solutions allow the forces to be determined to better than 95 percent accuracy (4). Such an approximation is not possible in analyzing the swing phase of gait or analyzing activities that involve large accelerations, such as throwing.

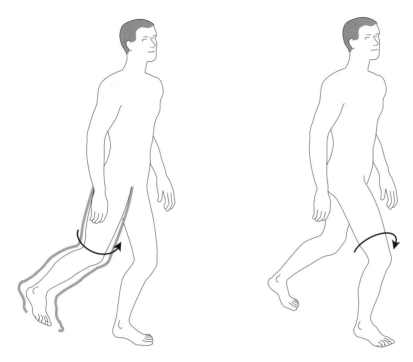

**Figure 1.16.** During gait, the thigh of the leg in stance phase rotates clockwise about the foot, and the thigh of the leg in swing phase rotates counterclockwise about the hip.

In these cases, the laws of dynamics must be utilized. To determine the forces and moments necessary to produce the observed dynamic performance of the limbs, we must apply the two fundamental principles of dynamics stated in Equations 1.1 and 1.2. To apply these principles, we must measure the accelerations and angular accelerations of each limb segment. We must also measure the mass and the mass moment of inertia of each of the segments. Then we can apply the dynamic equations and solve for the forces as products of the mass and acceleration, and the moments as products of the mass moment of inertia and the angular accelerations. For the musculoskeletal system, the force causing acceleration of the mass is the sum of muscle forces, joint reaction forces, gravity forces, and any external force. For example, in athletic endeavors such as the high jump, the ground reaction at takeoff acts as an external force.

The values of mass and mass moment of inertia for segments of the human body fortunately need not be determined in most cases. Extensive studies exist in the scientific literature and can be consulted to obtain these physical quantities (5). Measures of acceleration and angular acceleration are obtained from studies conducted on subjects in motion analysis laboratories (6). Each new clinical question may require observation to measure the accelerations and angular accelerations of the involved limb segments during the activity in question.

During studies of dynamic activities when the motion is observed, the external forces must also be determined. For activities such as walking, running, or jumping, the external force will be the reaction force of the ground pushing up on the feet. Ground reaction forces can be easily measured by force-sensing instruments (force plates) mounted in the floor on which the subject walks, runs, or jumps. For activities of the upper extremity, such as throwing a ball or swinging a tennis racket, the mass and mass moment of inertia of the object being thrown or swung must also be measured.

Let's examine an example of a dynamic problem. We will consider the force that must be exerted by the muscles about the hip joint at three different times during the swing phase of normal gait. Sequential positions of the lower limb during the swing phase are shown in Figure 1.16. The positions of the limb are observed at equal intervals of time. By knowing the time interval and measuring the angles of the limb segments at each position, the average angular velocity during the interval can be calculated (angular velocity equals the angle along the arc of motion between two successive positions divided by the time interval between the two positions). Then the angular acceleration can be determined from the change in angular velocity from one pair of observations to the next pair of observations (average angular acceleration equals the change in angular velocity between two pairs of observations divided by the time interval). The velocities and accelerations determined in this manner are shown in Figure 1.17.

We will assume that during the swing phase of gait the lower limb moves as a rigid body. This is a reasonable assumption, since the motion at the knee joint during swing phase is minimal. This assumption is important because it allows us to ignore any differences between the angular accelerations of the

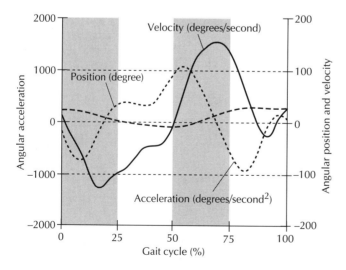

**Figure 1.17.** A plot of position, velocity, and acceleration for hip flexion and extension as a function of the phase of the gait cycle.

upper and lower leg, and because we need only worry about the mass properties of the entire limb. The mass properties of the lower limb can be obtained from the literature for the size and age of the subject being considered. For the subject in our problem, the mass moment of inertia is found to be $0.7 \text{ kg} \cdot \text{m}^2$ (5).

Equipped with the angular accelerations at each interval and the mass moment of inertia of the leg, we can now find the moment about the leg by applying the principle that the sum of the moments necessary to cause an observed angular acceleration of an object is equal to the mass moment of inertia of the object multiplied by the angular acceleration. There are two forces acting on the leg that can generate the moments necessary to produce the observed angular acceleration. One force that creates a moment is the gravity force acting on the mass of the leg. Note that the moment arm of this force about the center of rotation of the hip joint varies during the swing phase of the limb. The moment arm is longest at the beginning of the swing phase, when the hip is extended, and again at the end of the swing phase (just before heel strike), when the hip is flexed. At the middle of the swing phase, the moment arm of the gravity force is zero, since its line of action is vertical and will pass through the center of rotation of the hip joint.

The moment generated by the gravity force will have its maximum magnitudes, therefore, at the beginning and at the end of the swing phase. The magnitude of the moment will decrease to zero at the middle of the swing phase. Throughout the first half of the swing phase, while the hip joint is in extension, the moment created by the gravity force will tend to flex the hip joint; and throughout the second half of the swing phase, with the hip joint in flexion, the moment will tend to extend the hip joint.

The other force that creates a moment about the hip joint is the muscle force. The magnitude of the muscle force required to generate the moment will be equal to the magnitude of the moment divided by the muscle's moment arm about the hip joint. The muscles that tend to flex the hip joint will be active primarily during the first portion of the swing phase, as they angularly accelerate the leg. During the latter stages of the swing phase, the muscles that tend to extend the hip will be active, as they angularly decelerate the leg in preparation for heel strike.

Note the combined effect of the moment created by the gravity force and the moment created by these muscle actions. In the first half of the swing phase, the moment created by the gravity force tends to flex the hip, thus combining with the moment created by the hip flexor muscles to angularly accelerate the leg in flexion. The same is true in the latter half of the swing phase as the gravity force creates an ever-increasing moment in the opposite direction, aiding the moment created by the hip extensor muscles in angularly decelerating the swing of the limb in the direction of progression.

Let's consider the situation near the beginning of the swing phase, when the limb is angularly accelerating at 9 radians/second$^2$ (Fig. 1.16). For convenience, engineers and others in the physical sciences use a unit different from degrees to measure angles. The unit is a radian, and there are $2\pi$ radians in a full circle of 360 degrees. Therefore, *a radian is equal to approximately 57.3 degrees.* The radian is a convenient notation for angles because it allows the calculation of arc length about a circle in much simpler terms compared with the degree notation, as we will see in Chapter 2.

The moment required to produce the 9 radians/second$^2$ acceleration of the limb (with a mass moment of inertia of 0.7 kg $\cdot$ m$^2$) is (from Equation 1.2)

$$\text{Moment} = 0.7 \text{ kg} \cdot \text{m}^2 \times 9 \frac{\text{radians}}{\text{sec}^2}$$

$$\text{Moment} = 6.3 \frac{\text{kg} \cdot \text{m}^2}{\text{sec}^2} = 6.3 \text{ N} \cdot \text{m}$$

since a newton is defined as 1 kilogram-meter/second$^2$. This moment is the net moment created by the gravity force $(G)$ and the muscle force $(M)$. Both forces create moments that tend to flex the hip joint, so the net moment is the sum of the moments created by the gravity force and the muscle force:

$$\text{Moment} = (G \times d_G) + (M \times d_M)$$

where $d_G$ and $d_M$ are the moment arms of the gravity force and the muscle force, respectively.

The mass of the leg is 12 kilograms, so that the magnitude of the gravity force is 118 newtons. For the position of the limb we are considering, the moment arm of the gravity force is 0.15 meters. By observing the anatomy around the hip joint, we can determine the moment arm of the main hip flexor muscle, the iliopsoas, to be 0.03 meters. We can now substitute these values into the last equation and solve for the magnitude of the muscle force:

$$\text{Muscle force} = \frac{\text{Moment}}{G \times d_G} \times \frac{1}{d_M}$$

$$= \frac{6.3 \text{ N} \cdot \text{m}}{118 \text{ N} \times 0.15 \text{ m}} \times \frac{1}{0.03 \text{ m}}$$

$$= 11.9 \text{ N}$$

Thus, little muscle force is required to accelerate the leg in swing, because of the large moment provided by the gravity force.

### References

1. Crowninshield RD, Johnston RC, Andrews JG, Brand RA. A biomechanical investigation of the human hip. J Biomech 1978;11:75-85.
2. Cooney WP III, Chao EYS. Biomechanical analysis of static forces in the thumb during hand function. J Bone Joint Surg 1977;59A:27-36.
3. Crowninshield RD, Brand RA. A physiologically based criterion of muscle force prediction in locomotion. J Biomech 1981;14:793-801.

4. Patriarco AG, Mann RW, Simon SR, Mansour JM. An evaluation of the approaches of optimization models in the prediction of muscle forces during human gait. J Biomech 1981;14:513-525.

5. Braune W, Fischer O. Determination of the moments of inertia of the human body and its limbs. Berlin: Springer-Verlag, 1988.

6. Sutherland DH, Olshen RA, Biden EN, Wyatt MP. The development of mature walking. Oxford: Mac Keith Press, 1988.

# 2

## Musculoskeletal Performance

**WORK DUE TO FORCES**

**ENERGY STORAGE**

**WORK AND ENERGY DUE TO MOMENTS**

**POSITIVE AND NEGATIVE WORK**

**MEASUREMENT OF WORK EFFICIENCY**

**GAIT PERFORMANCE**

**JOINT MOMENTS CREATED BY
THE GROUND REACTION FORCE**

**DECELERATION-INDUCED NECK INJURY**

All organisms must perform work to survive in their environment. Work and the ability to do work (which we will call energy) must be incorporated into our understanding of the mechanical performance of living creatures. For example, it is necessary to do work and to expend energy when moving about on any type of surface. All muscles of the body, including the heart, are, in the simplest conception, machines that perform work. The skeletal system is the structure that transmits the work done by the muscles to the surrounding environment.

## WORK DUE TO FORCES

The concept of work is used to quantify certain specific activities. For example, if a man has climbed a flight of stairs, as shown in Figure 2.1, one measure of the activity is that the man has gained 3 meters of elevation. Muscle activity and the associated chemical changes were required for the man to achieve this performance. The mechanical description of the activity is that the man raised his weight a vertical distance of 3 meters, while also moving his weight forward a horizontal distance of 4 meters. Clearly, a different intensity of muscle activity was associated with the 3-meter increase in vertical distance as opposed to the 4-meter forward progression. This difference is best described by the concept of work.

In mechanical terms, *work can be defined as the moving of a force through a distance*. The force and the distance the force moves must be in the same direction. For example, in our stair-climbing illustration, the force that is moving the person is the ground reaction force pushing upward against the weight of the body. This ground reaction force must move upward 3 meters and forward 4 meters. In the upward motion, the direction of the force coincides with the direction of its motion. The work done by the force in this instance is calculated as the product of the force multiplied by the distance moved in the direction of the force:

$$\text{Work} = \text{Force} \times \text{Distance} \qquad (2.1)$$

For the forward motion, the direction in which the ground reaction force moves is perpendicular to the direction of the force. This action requires no work. Though this seems complicated, the concepts are actually intuitive. One can coast on a bicycle, for example, with no muscle activity. The less wind resistance and friction acting to slow the bicycle, the longer the distance traveled. In this case, the reaction force caused by the wheel contacting the ground is also directed upward, that is, perpendicular to the direction of travel. But no work is required to move the reaction force in the horizontal direction. However, a bicycle cannot coast uphill. The wheel contact force has a vertical component, and to raise this force component in the vertical direction as the bike climbs the hill requires work.

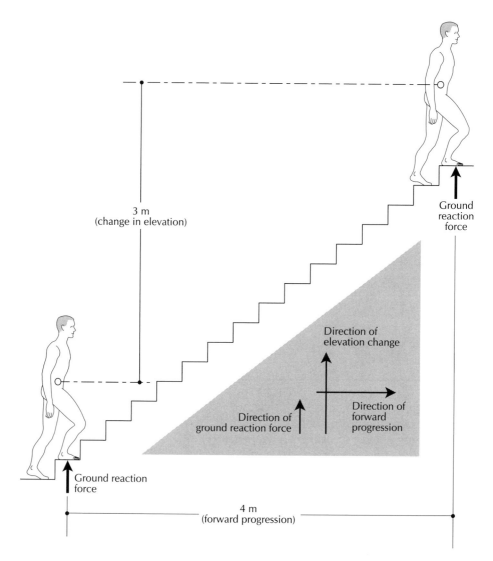

**Figure 2.1.** By use of muscle action, a person climbing the steps would experience a change in elevation of 3 meters while progressing in the forward direction 4 meters. The muscle activity associated with the elevation change differs greatly from that associated with the forward progression.

Consider the action of the muscle contraction of the patient undergoing leg rehabilitation on an exercise machine (Fig. 1.15). If, instead of an isometric effort, we allow the machine to turn about the center of rotation of the axle, the hamstring muscles exert a force on the tibia, and that force is directed along the line of action of the hamstring muscles (Fig. 2.2). As the muscles contract, they move the force acting on the tibia in the same direction as the line of action of the force. Because the muscles have moved the point of application of their contractile force, the muscles have done work. The amount of work is equal to the muscles' force multiplied by the distance that the force moved.

In general, when muscles contract, the direction of movement of the muscle's contractile force is coincident with the direction of the muscle force. If a weight lifter is to dead-lift 200 kilograms of mass through a distance of 0.75 meters, his hands must exert a vertically directed force equal to the weight of the 200-kilogram mass (Fig. 2.3). This force will be

$$\text{Force} = 200 \text{ kg} \times 9.8 \text{ m/sec}^2$$
$$= 1960 \text{ N}$$

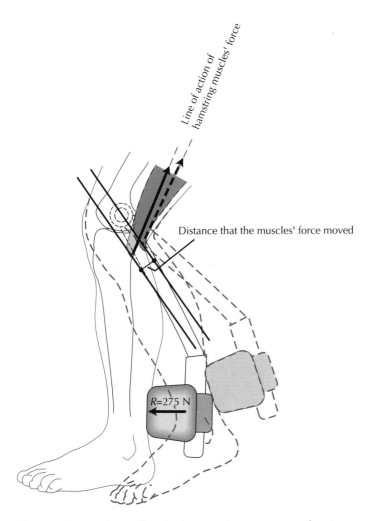

**Figure 2.2.** In order to flex the knee against an external resistance, the hamstring muscles must contract (shorten their length). The contracted muscles' force, as it moves with the flexing leg, performs work on the leg.

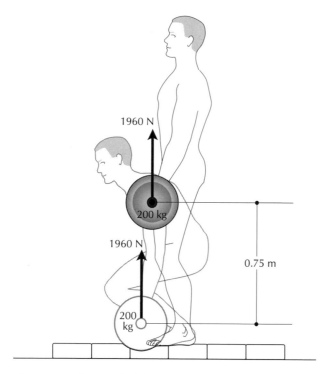

**Figure 2.3.** The weight lifter raises a 200-kilogram mass to a distance of three-quarters of a meter. The amount of work he performs is equal to the weight of the mass multiplied by the height change of the center of gravity of the mass.

The force exerted by the hands must travel through the 0.75 meters to raise the barbell. The weight lifter must therefore produce an amount of work (from Equation 2.1) equal to

$$\text{Work} = 1960 \text{ N} \times 0.75 \text{ m}$$

$$= 1470 \text{ N} \cdot \text{m}$$

$$= 1470 \text{ J}$$

Note that in Chapter 1 we described moments in units of newton-meters. The concept of a moment, however, does not involve motion of the force; it is a static effect. This is contrasted with the concept of work, which involves motion of the force. In the international system of units, *a joule (J) equals the work performed by a force of 1 newton moving through a distance of 1 meter.*

## ENERGY STORAGE

Closely associated with the concept of work is the concept of energy. *Energy is the ability to perform work.* Therefore, intrinsically associated with energy is the concept of storage. Work is the result of the release of energy. Biological organisms store energy in chemical form. When required to do work (that is, to contract a muscle), the organism releases chemical energy and transforms it to a muscle contraction. The muscle contraction then performs mechanical work.

There are many forms in which energy is stored, and each is described by a specific adjective. We have already mentioned chemical energy, which is the most important form in which organisms store energy. Other forms of energy storage include potential energy, kinetic energy, and strain energy.

*Potential energy is energy stored by virtue of a weight being raised above a reference plane.* When the weight lifter raised the 200-kilogram (mass) barbell, the work done in lifting the weight was actually stored in the barbell. This can be easily observed if you realize that the barbell has the ability to perform work if it is lowered to the floor mat. The barbell can exert a force of 1960 newtons directed vertically downward during the entire traverse of 0.75 meters from the raised position back down to the mat. Thus, in the lowering of the barbell, the barbell itself performs work on the weight lifter. This is in contrast to the lifting of the barbell, where the weight lifter had to perform work on the barbell.

At the raised position, the barbell has the potential of doing work in an amount equal to the weight multiplied by its height above the mat. In fact, any weight raised above a reference plane has potential energy:

$$\text{Potential energy} = \text{Weight} \times \text{Height} \qquad (2.2)$$

Suppose the weight lifter chose not to lower the barbell, but to drop it instead. Let's examine the energy in the barbell at the moment before it strikes the mat. The barbell will no longer possess potential energy, because it no longer has any height above the mat. It will, however, have velocity in the vertical direction. Because of this velocity, the barbell will have the ability to push against the floor mat while the mat pushes up to stop the fall of the barbell. The resulting deformation in the mat as the barbell lands on it means that the barbell has done work against the floor mat.

The barbell, therefore, at the instant before impact with the mat, *has energy by virtue of its velocity. This type of energy is called kinetic energy.* Kinetic energy is calculated as follows:

$$\text{Kinetic energy} = \frac{1}{2} \times \text{Mass} \times \text{Velocity}^2 \qquad (2.3)$$

Where did this kinetic energy originate? It comes from the potential energy in the barbell just before it is released. The amount of kinetic energy in the barbell just before it strikes the mat is equal to the amount of potential energy the barbell possessed before it was dropped. The potential energy of the barbell is (from Equation 2.2)

$$\text{Potential energy} = 1960 \text{ N} \times 0.75 \text{ m}$$
$$= 1470 \text{ J}$$

To calculate the kinetic energy, we must determine the velocity of the barbell just before it strikes the mat. For a free-falling object accelerating under the influence of gravity,

$$\text{Velocity}^2 = 2 \times \text{Acceleration of gravity} \times \text{Distance} \qquad (2.4)$$

Considering that the barbell falls through a distance of 0.75 meters, accelerating due to gravity at 9.8 m/sec$^2$, the velocity can be calculated from Equation 2.4:

$$\text{Velocity}^2 = 2 \times 9.8 \ \frac{\text{m}}{\text{sec}^2} \times 0.75 \ \text{m}$$

$$= 14.7 \ \frac{\text{m}^2}{\text{sec}^2}$$

$$\text{Velocity} = \sqrt{14.7 \frac{\text{m}^2}{\text{sec}^2}}$$

$$= 3.834 \ \text{m/sec}$$

The kinetic energy of the barbell just before it strikes the mat (from Equation 2.3) is

$$\text{Kinetic energy} = \frac{1}{2} \times 200 \ \text{kg} \times \left(3.834 \ \frac{\text{m}}{\text{sec}}\right)^2$$

$$= 1470 \ \text{m} \cdot \frac{\text{kg} \cdot \text{m}}{\text{sec}^2}$$

Remember that 1 kilogram-meter/second$^2$ is a newton.

When the barbell does strike the floor mat, the mat deforms and pushes back up on the barbell, stopping its motion. The barbell in turn pushes down on the mat, causing it to deform, thus doing work on the mat. When the mat is deformed, it possesses the ability of springing back to its original shape, even to the extent of pushing the heavy barbell slightly upward. *The ability of a structure to do work by virtue of its being deformed is called strain energy* and is dealt with more thoroughly in Chapter 4. For our current purposes, it is sufficient to think of strain energy as energy that is stored in a spring when the spring is deformed (Fig. 2.4). To compress the spring, we allow the barbell to rest on the spring and do work against the resistance of the spring. The spring has the ability to do work against the barbell if we raise the barbell and allow the spring to expand to its original shape. Therefore, in its compressed position, the spring has the ability to do work by virtue of its deformed shape.

As another example of the role played by energy, consider a traumatic event such as a fall. A standing person possesses potential energy by virtue of the person's weight being at a higher level compared with a second position (Fig. 2.5). The center of gravity in the first position is 0.8 meters above the ground, while the center of gravity in the second position is only 0.3 meters above the

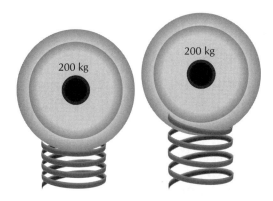

**Figure 2.4.** When a 200-kilogram mass is lowered onto a spring, it compresses the spring. The 1960-newton gravity force (weight) of the mass is lowered as it contacts the spring, and the mass thus gives up potential energy. Some of this potential energy is stored in the spring.

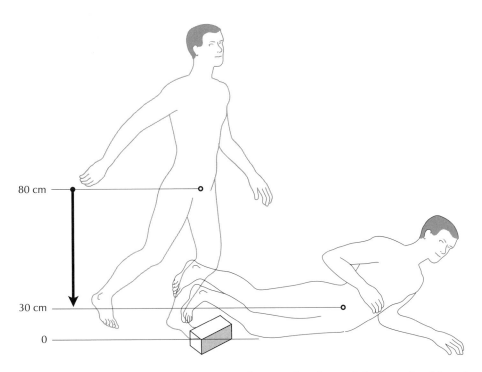

**Figure 2.5.** A standing person has potential energy by virtue of the fact that his or her center of gravity is above the floor. If the person falls, the center of gravity is suddenly lowered. The potential energy is then converted to kinetic energy, and at the point of impact the kinetic energy must be absorbed within the body of the person falling and in the surface upon which he or she fell.

ground. The individual's weight is 700 newtons. The difference in potential energy between the two positions can be calculated as

$$\text{Potential energy} = (700 \text{ N} \times 0.8 \text{ m}) - (700 \text{ N} \times 0.3 \text{ m})$$
$$= 350 \text{ J}$$

In the case of a fall, all the potential energy will be converted to kinetic energy by the time the person makes contact with the ground. At the moment of contact, the kinetic energy will be absorbed by both the person's hip and the ground. This energy absorption will deform both the hip and the ground, causing strain energy to be developed in both of these structures. If the magnitude of the strain energy created in the hip is large, the bony structures in the hip may not remain intact.

## WORK AND ENERGY DUE TO MOMENTS

The concept of work involves moving a force through a distance, with the direction of the force and the direction of the motion of the force being the same. But what happens when the force moves along a curved path? Let's consider a simple example where the force moves along a circular pathway (Fig. 2.6). We will apply a 150-newton force to a 10-meter lever arm to move it against the resistance at the pivot point of the lever. The force will move the arm through an angle of 20 degrees. Since at every point along the circular path, both the force and the motion of the force are tangent to the path, the work will still be equal to the force multiplied by the distance through which the force moves.

The force moves through a 20-degree or 0.349-radian circular arc. As mentioned in Chapter 1, using the radian as a unit of angular measurement allows easy calculation of the length of a circular arc. *The length of any arc is simply the radius of the arc's circle multiplied by the arc's angle (in radians).* The distance the force moves in our example is therefore

$$\text{Distance} = \text{Arc length}$$
$$= \text{Radius} \times \text{Angle (radians)} \tag{2.5}$$

The work done by the force moving through the 0.349-radian angle is therefore

$$\text{Work} = \text{Force} \times \text{Radius} \times \text{Angle}$$
$$= 150 \text{ N} \times 10 \text{ m} \times 0.349 \text{ radians}$$
$$= 523.5 \text{ J}$$

But the force multiplied by the radius is the moment produced by the force about the pivot point of the lever arm. Thus, in calculating the work done by the force in causing the arm to rotate, it is equivalent to use

$$\text{Work} = \text{Moment} \times \text{Angle} \tag{2.6}$$

where the angle is measured in radians.

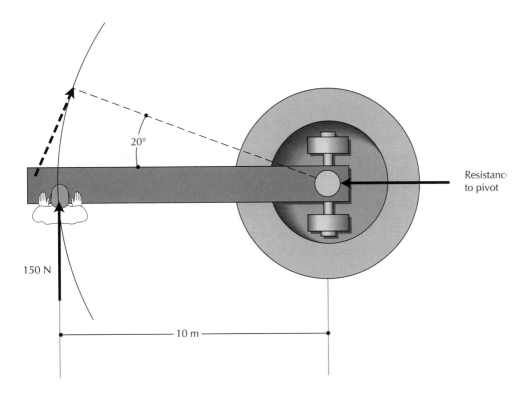

**Figure 2.6.** A person pushes against a rotating lever with a force of 150 newtons. The point of application of the force moves along a circular pathway. The work performed by the person may be calculated either as the applied force multiplied by the length of the arc through which the force moves, or by the applied moment (150 newtons multiplied by 10 meters) multiplied by the angle through which the moment moves.

Consider another example involving the exercise machine. Instead of isokinetic exercise (Fig. 2.2), the patient performs isotonic exercise, with the machine providing a moment-resisting rotation at the knee joint of 50 newton-meters. When the patient flexes the knee through an angle of 75 degrees (1.31 radians) against this resistance, the work done by the hamstring muscles in moving the arm of the machine will be (from Equation 2.6)

$$\text{Work} = 50\ \text{N} \cdot \text{m} \times 1.31\ \text{radians}$$
$$= 65.5\ \text{J}$$

## POSITIVE AND NEGATIVE WORK

A muscle can perform work by shortening while it exerts a force against its attachment points. But a biological counterpart exists in which the muscle also exerts force against its attachment points while those points are separating.

When the attachment points of a muscle come closer together (concentric muscle contraction), the muscle does work on the skeleton. When the attachment points separate (eccentric muscle contraction), the skeleton is doing work on the muscle. The first case, in which the muscle does the work, is called *positive muscle work*. The second case, in which the muscle has work done to it, is called *negative muscle work*.

The biomechanical importance of concentric contraction of muscles is that it allows people to move about, to lift objects, to climb structures, and to operate tools and machinery. The biomechanical importance of eccentric contraction of muscles is that it allows people to descend stairs, lower a weight to the ground, and absorb energy in a fall.

When a muscle undergoes an eccentric contraction, little of the negative muscle work is stored within the muscle itself. Except near full extension of the muscle, most of the work is dissipated. Muscles can absorb large quantities of energy during eccentric contraction, because they can exert large forces throughout a large excursion.

## MEASUREMENT OF WORK EFFICIENCY

All animals live by virtue of the conversion of chemical energy into mechanical energy. Parallel processes of cell rejuvenation and growth and the metabolism of food products to convert stored chemical energy to heat are both dependent on the mechanical circulation of blood and air. The mechanical processes performed during the activities of daily living have, therefore, an associated energy cost. This cost is composed of two parts: that part directly associated with the activity (for example, walking) and that part associated with maintaining homeostasis (for example, breathing, blood circulation, maintaining body temperature, and nourishing cells).

Because all conversion of energy within the body starts with the oxidation of nutrients, the metabolism of the body can be monitored by measuring the quantities of oxygen (and carbon dioxide) in the inhaled and expired air. For example, the amount of energy expenditure by a resting man is approximately 17 calories/minute/kilogram of body mass. This corresponds to the use of oxygen at the rate of approximately 3.4 milliliters of oxygen/minute/kilogram of body mass (1). This can be contrasted with a person walking at a natural, freely chosen speed (usually called the free velocity) of approximately 80 meters/minute. The person will consume about 12 milliliters of oxygen/minute/kilogram of body mass. A useful measure of the efficiency of walking is the energy expended to travel 1 meter. This description of energy expenditure is analogous to the description of gas "mileage" for an automobile. If the gas "mileage" is divided by the mass of the car, we can obtain an exact analogy in terms of liters per kilometer traveled per kilogram.

An average male walking at the free speed of 80 meters/minute consumes 0.15 milliliters of oxygen/meter/kilogram. When a person tries to walk faster or slower than his or her free velocity, the energy cost tends to increase markedly (1). Since humans do not walk fast enough to consider wind resistance a significant factor influencing energy efficiency, what other causes could there be for this phenomenon? In Chapter 1 we showed that gravity helps to accelerate and decelerate the leg during the swing phase of gait. If we try to move our legs faster or slower than the natural rhythm produced by gravity (comparable to a swinging pendulum), we require larger muscle forces to provide increased flexion moment at the hip joint to accelerate the leg at the start of the swing phase, and increased extension moment at the end of the swing phase to decelerate the leg. A similar situation exists for slow walking. Larger muscle forces are required to decrease the acceleration of the leg at the start of the swing phase and to decrease deceleration at terminal swing. Thus, the increases in energy expenditure and the oxygen consumption rate at slow or fast walking speeds result from the need for increased muscle activity as compared with walking at the free speed.

Similarly, any disability resulting in an asymmetry of gait will result in an increase in the mechanical energy required for gait. Consider a patient with right-foot pain walking at a "normal" free velocity. To limit the pain, the patient shortens the stance time on the right leg and lengthens the stance time on the pain-free left leg. The swing phase of the right leg will of necessity take more time, and this will require muscle control similar to the pattern of slow gait that we just described. The left leg will have a shorter swing phase, similar to the pattern of rapid gait. Each of the altered swing activities imposes additional energy costs. Therefore, even though the patient is walking at a "normal" free velocity, the swing phase of each leg behaves in a manner that increases the energy cost. Other causes for increased oxygen consumption include deviations from normal limb structure and lack of functional muscle control over limb segments. For example, increased oxygen consumption has been measured in patients with asymptomatic congenital dislocation of the hip and in patients with an artificial limb segment (2). In both cases, increased muscle force is required in at least a portion of the limb to provide the necessary motion control. The increased muscle forces produce increased work and, hence, increased energy expenditure.

Since the goal in many rehabilitative procedures is to restore a more normal gait pattern in the patient, the rate of oxygen consumption can be used as a sensitive indicator of the degree of normalcy. It is accepted that a person may walk without limit if the rate of energy expenditure does not exceed 50 percent of the person's aerobic capacity. Therefore, those treatments that allow the patient to maintain an energy expenditure below this limit can, in an absolute sense, be considered satisfactory if the criterion of unlimited ambulation is accepted.

## GAIT PERFORMANCE

The biomechanical analysis of gait is useful at several levels of understanding. Ambulation is one of the most important of human functions, and the degradation of a person's ambulatory capacity often requires medical treatment. While much information about the quality of gait can be derived from simple observation, we will deal here with those aspects that can be quantified by measurement or analysis.

A functional description of gait is that activity that allows an individual to move from position A to position B while maintaining the body in a generally upright and stable posture. The mechanics of gait can be thought of as a force application system between the ground and the individual's feet that drives the body along its intended pathway. Coupled with this force control system between the ground and the feet is a postural force control system that maintains the desired upright posture of the trunk and head. We will consider only the control system associated with the ground reaction force.

The ground reaction force has three major functions: to maintain the progression of motion in the desired direction, to minimize motion of the body perpendicular to the direction of progression, and to maintain the center of gravity of the body at as constant a height as possible. This last function acts to minimize the energy cost of gait, since raising and lowering the center of gravity of the body during each step requires energy expenditure that does not contribute to moving the body forward.

Let's analyze the forces and moments associated with each of these three functions. Forward motion is initiated by changing the forward component of the velocity. This forward acceleration requires a net ground reaction force in the forward direction acting on the feet. When the person starts walking at a free velocity of 80 meters/minute (1.33 meters/second), a change in velocity from 0 meters/second to 1.33 meters/second over a period of one-quarter of a second is observed. A net horizontal force will be required equal to the mass of the body multiplied by the average acceleration. The average acceleration will be the change in velocity (1.33 meters/second) divided by the time over which the change in velocity occurs (0.25 seconds). For a person with a body mass of 70 kilograms, the required force will be (from Equation 1.1)

$$\text{Force} = 70 \text{ kg} \times \frac{1.33 \text{ m/sec}}{0.25 \text{ sec}}$$

$$= 372 \text{ N}$$

After the acceleration, the body continues to move forward at a constant velocity. Since there is no further acceleration in the forward direction, the net force acting on the foot over the gait cycle in the forward direction will be zero, until the person stops or changes direction. This means that the anteriorly directed ground reaction force at toe-off, averaged over time, added to the posteriorly directed ground reaction force occurring at heel strike, averaged over the same time period, will sum to zero.

A plot of the force-versus-time history of the forward and aft horizontal components of the ground reaction force taken during the constant-velocity portion of a patient's gait study is shown in Figure 2.7. The average anteriorly directed force will be equal to the area under the force-versus-time plot divided by the time of application. The same is true for the posteriorly directed force. If we compare these two areas, we will observe that they are equal, meaning

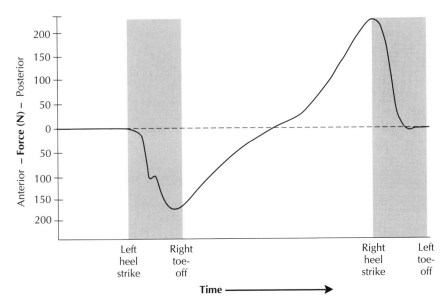

**Figure 2.7.** The forward and aft horizontal components of the ground reaction force were recorded during the stance phase of gait. Even though the subject walked at constant velocity, the component of the ground reaction force in the horizontal direction has both forward and aft components. The average force for each limb is zero.

that the average anterior-posterior force is zero. For normal gait this is true for both legs individually.

The same argument can be applied to the limited change in velocity in the medial-lateral direction when the subject is walking in a straight line. Over a complete gait cycle, the average force for both limbs in this direction must be zero (Fig. 2.8). Consider the right leg of a patient. The medial-lateral forces show a marked asymmetry, because the patient must exert a medially directed force to first stop the motion of the center of gravity of the body toward the right side and then move it toward the left side in time for the stance phase of the left limb. This medially directed force is counterbalanced by a laterally directed force when the center of gravity is returned to its position over the right leg for the next cycle. Notice also the magnitudes of the medial-lateral forces for both legs. These are the force components that create varus and valgus moments about the ankle, knee, and hip joints.

Efficient gait requires that the vertical motion of the body's center of gravity between steps be minimized. Any muscle effort that raises the center of gravity may be wasted when the center of gravity is subsequently lowered. There are compensating mechanisms that can save some of this energy, but they involve speeding up and slowing down the movement of the center of gravity. Thus, as you raise your center of gravity during the initial part of the stance phase of gait, you decrease your forward velocity slightly. Likewise, as you lower your center of gravity during the terminal part of the stance phase, you increase your forward velocity slightly (3).

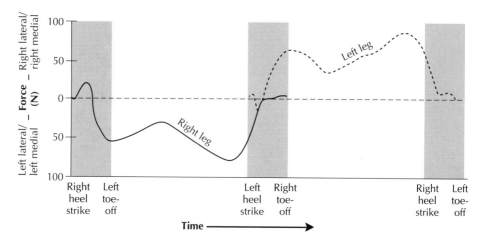

**Figure 2.8.** At the same time that the forward and aft horizontal components of the ground reaction force were measured (Fig. 2.7), the medial-lateral forces were also recorded. The person walked in a straight line, but nevertheless there are components of the ground reaction force in both the medial and lateral directions. The average force for both limbs is zero.

## JOINT MOMENTS CREATED
## BY THE GROUND REACTION FORCE

We have considered the ground reaction force imposed upon the foot during the stance phase of gait to be composed of three mutually orthogonal components when analyzing vertical, forward, or lateral motion. In examining moments about the hip, knee, and ankle joints, we may wish to visualize the ground reaction force as a single vector (the sum of the components) in space originating at the center of contact between the foot and the ground and extending out into space in the general direction of the stance limb. During walking, the ground reaction force usually varies from about 0.85 times body weight to about 1.15 times body weight in magnitude. It is thus much larger than the gravity force that acts directly on the lower limb (approximately one-sixth of body weight). If we want to obtain an approximation of the moment imposed on either the ankle, knee, or hip joint, we may ignore the limb gravity force and only consider the moment produced by the ground reaction force about any of these joints.

During the initial portion of the stance phase, the ground reaction force passes posterior and lateral to the knee joint (Fig. 2.9). Thus, to prevent the knee from collapsing, both an extension moment and a varus moment must be generated at the knee joint. The extension moment is created by the quadriceps muscle pulling on its attachment point on the tibia through the patellar ligament. If, at this instant in the gait cycle, the line of action of the ground reaction force is located 0.1 meters behind the center of rotation of the knee joint and its magnitude is 700 newtons, the resulting flexion moment will be 70 newton-meters. To counterbalance this moment with an extension moment of equal magnitude, the force created in the patellar ligament, acting at a distance of 0.05 meters from the contact point in the knee joint, must equal

$$\text{Force}_{\text{Pat Lig}} = \frac{70 \text{ N} \cdot \text{m}}{0.05 \text{ m}}$$

$$= 1400 \text{ N}$$

The valgus moment created by the ground reaction force is counterbalanced by a varus moment created by the joint contact force (see Chapter 3, page 75).

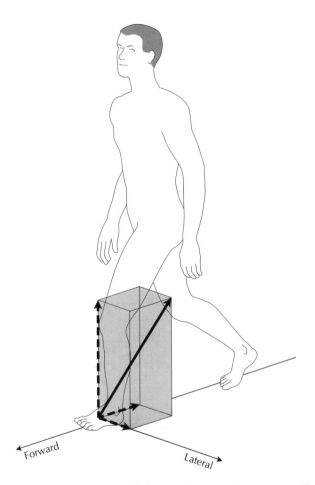

**Figure 2.9.** The ground reaction force at this point in the gait cycle produces a flexion moment at the knee because it passes behind the knee's center of rotation.

**Figure 2.10.** Attempting to make a tackle, the defensive player impacts with the top of his helmet against the leg of the ball carrier.

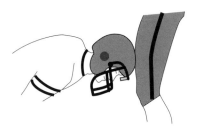

## DECELERATION-INDUCED NECK INJURY

Acceleration and deceleration of the trunk is usually accomplished by relatively slow application of moderate force. This is true in activities including high-performance athletics, such as track and field. Contact sports, however, offer occasions during which the forces applied to accelerate and decelerate the trunk can result in severe skeletal injury. A notorious example is cervical spine injury occurring in football during head-first tackles (4). This same injury can result from diving into shallow water, where head-first contact with the ground may occur. Hockey players who slide head first into the sideboards have also been victims of this mechanism of injury. The injury mechanism in these cases results from the forces generated in the cervical spine to decelerate the trunk.

Consider a defensive back who is making a tackle on a ball carrier (Fig. 2.10). At the moment of impact, the back has lowered his head and eliminated the lordotic curve of the cervical spine. He makes contact with the crown of his helmet against the thigh pad of the ball carrier. The tackler is moving at approximately 5 meters per second at impact, with the ball carrier moving at about the same velocity. In the sequence of events that follows over the next 20 milliseconds, the tackler's helmet first comes to a stop, followed about 3 or 4 milliseconds later by the tackler's head.

The distance over which the head stops its forward motion is approximately 3 centimeters, that is, the distance that the padding in the helmet can compress. To calculate the average force required to stop the head, we can use Equation 2.4. We know the stopping distance (0.03 meters) and the loss in velocity over that distance (5 meters/second), so we can calculate the average deceleration:

$$\text{Average deceleration} = \frac{\text{Velocity}^2}{2 \times \text{Distance}}$$

$$= \frac{(5 \text{ m}/\text{sec})^2}{2 \times 0.03 \text{ m}}$$

$$= 417 \text{ m}/\text{sec}^2$$

We can now calculate the average force required to decelerate the head. The mass of the head is approximately 5 kilograms. Using Equation 1.1, the average force is the mass of the head multiplied by the average deceleration:

$$\text{Average force} = 5 \text{ kg} \times 417 \text{ m/sec}^2$$

$$= 2085 \text{ N}$$

When the head has slowed substantially, the skull restricts the motion of the first cervical vertebra, which in turn is being pushed toward the head by the remaining cervical vertebrae. The seventh cervical vertebra (C-7), while being impeded by C-6, is also being pushed toward the head by the trunk. This produces a compressive force on C-7, since it is tending to move slower than the trunk. Conversely, a force is generated by C-7 on the trunk to decelerate the trunk's velocity.

The head is provided a stopping distance of 3 centimeters by virtue of the padding in the helmet. The cervical spine can compress about 2 centimeters when placed in a straight position before it will buckle and suffer acute local hyperflexion. This gives the trunk a total stopping distance of only 5 centimeters before injury to the cervical spine will occur. Compressing the cervical spine 2 centimeters requires a force of about 5000 newtons. Any higher force level will cause failure of either a disc or a vertebral body and will result in buckling of the cervical column.

Let's determine what the change in the velocity of the trunk will be as the trunk moves a distance of 5 centimeters, during which time the cervical spine provides an average stopping force of 2500 newtons. We arrive at the average stopping force by averaging the maximum force that the cervical spine can produce (5000 newtons) and the initial force value (0 newtons). The mass of the tackler's trunk is 35 kilograms. Using Equation 1.1, the average deceleration of the trunk is equal to the average stopping force for the trunk divided by the mass of the trunk:

$$\text{Average deceleration} = \frac{2500 \text{ N}}{35 \text{ kg}}$$

$$= 71.4 \text{ m/sec}^2$$

This average deceleration produced during the time the trunk is moving a distance of 5 centimeters will cause a decrease in velocity (from Equation 2.4) of

$$\text{Velocity}^2 = 2 \times 71.4 \text{ m/sec}^2 \times 0.05 \text{ m}$$

$$= 7.14 \text{ m}^2/\text{sec}^2$$

$$\text{Average decrease in velocity} = 2.7 \text{ m/sec}$$

Thus, by the time the cervical spine is compressed its maximum amount without sustaining injury, the trunk has lost only about half of its velocity. In addition, the ball carrier still has a substantial portion of his velocity remaining. This means that the trunk will continue to compress the cervical spine beyond its critical point with catastrophic consequences.

## *References*

1. Inman VT, Ralston HJ, Todd F. Human walking. Baltimore: Williams & Wilkins, 1981:62-69.
2. Otis JC, Lane JM, Kroll MA. Energy cost during gait in osteosarcoma patients after resection and knee replacement and after above-the-knee amputation. J Bone Joint Surg 1985;67A:606-611.
3. Inman VT, Ralston HJ, Todd F. Human walking. Baltimore: Williams & Wilkins, 1981:39.
4. Otis JC, Burstein AH, Torg JS. Mechanisms and pathomechanics of athletic injuries to the cervical spine. In: Torg JS, ed. Athletic injuries to the head, neck, and face. 2nd ed. St. Louis: Mosby Year Book, 1991:438-456.

# 3

## Joint Stability

**DEFINITIONS OF JOINT STABILITY**
**MECHANISMS OF JOINT STABILITY**
**STABILITY IN NORMAL AND ABNORMAL JOINTS**
**STABILITY IN JOINTS WITH LIGAMENTOUS INJURIES**

## DEFINITIONS OF JOINT STABILITY

### Joint Stability in the Plane of Motion

Since the function of the musculoskeletal system is to provide control of motion, any factor affecting motion of diarthrodial joints can have a critical effect on skeletal performance. The concept of joint stability is intimately associated with the concept of joint motion. *The most general definition of joint stability is the ability of a joint to maintain an appropriate functional position throughout its range of motion.* Thus, a joint is stable if, when moving through a normal range of motion, it can carry the required functional loads without pain and produce joint contact forces of normal intensity on its articular cartilage surfaces.

Stable joints are characterized by several key functions. Joint contact occurs between surfaces covered with articular cartilage. Peripheral or edge loading does not seem to occur in normal, stable joints. Stable joints have one position of joint equilibrium for any particular functional loading situation. The application of small additional increments of functional load does not produce sudden, large changes in the position of joint contact. Similarly, small changes in the direction of the functional load do not produce large, sudden changes in joint contact position. Thus, if a knee joint is supporting a flexion moment, an applied small tibial torque should not produce a sudden, large angular displacement.

### Joint Stability in the Lateral Plane

Some joints, such as the hip joint, exhibit gross motion in planes of nearly all directions. Other joints, such as the knee joint, provide motion in a dominant direction, such as the plane of progression. Our definition of joint stability applies to all of these directions of motion. However, similar concepts of stability apply in directions other than the dominant direction. For example, the knee joint has a large measurable range of motion for flexion and extension, but not for varus and valgus angulation or internal and external rotation. Therefore, we can modify our previous concept of stability in the plane of motion for application to the lateral plane. *In this plane, a stable joint is one that maintains an appropriate minimum contact force between the articulating surfaces throughout the functional range of motion of the joint. Joint stability is the ability to control both lateral translations and rotations, so as to maintain contact on nonperipheral, centrally located regions of the articular cartilage while still allowing functional control in the normal plane of motion.*

Our definitions of stability now allow us to recognize unstable joints. A knee joint that cannot move into full flexion because of a large, abnormal posterior motion of the tibia relative to the femur is unstable. A knee joint that cannot fully flex because the tibia has rotated in an abnormal manner is unstable. A patella whose central region contacts the lateral border of the femoral groove during flexion is also unstable.

## MECHANISMS OF JOINT STABILITY

### Mechanisms in the Plane of Motion

The most passive mechanism of joint constraint that provides stability is the control of the location of the joint contact force by the curvature of the articular contact surfaces. As we noted in Chapter 1 (page 11), contact between two articular surfaces results in compressive forces that are aligned at 90 degrees to the contact surfaces. Because of the extremely low coefficient of friction between articular surfaces, the perpendicular alignment of the contact force and the contact surface exists whether the joint is stationary or moving. As we also observed in Chapter 1, for any particular functional loading situation, the direction of the joint reaction force is controlled by the magnitude and the direction of the functional load and by the magnitude and the direction of the necessary responding muscle force. Thus, for every activity (see Figs. 1.12B, 1.14, and 1.15), there exists a functional load and a corresponding muscle force that together require a particular magnitude and orientation of joint reaction force.

We will now determine how that joint reaction force is produced. The simplest and most direct way to produce joint reaction force is by compression of two articular joint surfaces. In Figure 3.1A, we show a hypothetical joint and the required joint reaction force. We ask, can this joint produce the required joint reaction force by joint compression alone? To determine the answer, we note in Figure 3.1B that in moving the superior portion of the joint from position I to position II, we have included all possible stable contact regions according to our previous definition of joint stability. In Figure 3.1C, we have constructed lines that are perpendicular to the joint surfaces at the extremes of the range of stable joint contact. At these extreme positions, the joint surfaces are capable of producing joint contact forces in the indicated directions. These directions are, of course, perpendicular to the joint surfaces at the point of contact. These two directions represent limits of the envelope of all possible orientations of joint contact forces. Examination of our required joint contact force shows that it falls within the limits of the two extreme directions. Thus, if we orient the joint surfaces as in Figure 3.1D, the contact point (p) allows a joint compression force that matches the required joint reaction direction. We can now achieve equilibrium by a joint reaction that is created by only a joint compression force. The joint is operating in a stable fashion, since it fulfills all of our requirements for stability.

This example shows a joint stabilized by the curvature of its contact surfaces. Note that this is a passive mechanism. The joint curvature cannot be rapidly or voluntarily changed. The joint involuntarily seeks a contact position consistent with the production of an appropriately directed joint reaction force. If the joint undergoes a small motion with no abrupt changes in functional load, then the resulting small changes in the direction of the joint reaction force will produce small movements of the joint surfaces as they seek to establish contact at the appropriate position along the radius of curvature.

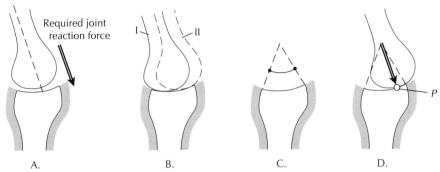

Figure 3.1. *A.* The joint must produce the joint reaction force shown. The flexion angle must remain constant. *B.* For the required angle of flexion the joint can assume any stable position between position I and position II. *C.* The range of orientation of the joint reaction force that can be produced by joint contact alone is shown. *D.* The joint will seek the contact position where the perpendicular to the contacting surfaces at the contact point (*p*) is in the required direction.

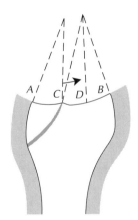

**Figure 3.2.** A joint with a discontinuity is shown. The range of orientation is bounded by lines *A* and *B*. If the joint contact at position *C* is altered slightly, a large motion of the contacting surface from *C* to *D* will result. The orientation at position *D* is only slightly different from the orientation at position *C*.

Joints that have been subjected to a transarticular fracture and, therefore, that may have abrupt changes of the surface curvature, may not be stable. Figure 3.2 illustrates a joint that has healed after a compression fracture altered the normal joint curvature. The total range of orientation of the joint reaction force still extends from position *A* to position *B*. However, if during a functional cycle the motion of the joint reaction force requires the orientation of the joint reaction force to move from position *C* to position *D*, the joint surfaces will undergo a sudden motion as the contact surfaces jump from *C* to *D*. We see that even though the joint has contiguous surfaces, small changes in the joint surface associated with a cusp or surface discontinuity can still produce an unstable joint. In this case, the instability is associated with large or sudden changes in joint position due to small or gradual changes in functional load.

The amount of stability provided by the curvature of the joint surface varies greatly among joints. The hip joint can provide compressive forces throughout the large range of orientation of required joint reaction forces because of the large included angle of the acetabulum. While the shoulder joint is analogous to the hip joint with respect to its range of motion, the range of orientation of the compressive joint contact force is much more limited because of the rather small included angle of the glenoid.

Most static loading situations produce joint reaction forces that can be provided by joint compressive loading. This mechanism is so effective partly because of the geometry of the attachment of muscles spanning the joint. As an example, consider the knee joint in its fully flexed, partially flexed, and fully extended positions (Fig. 3.3). One of the two joint surfaces, the tibial plateau, has a much smaller variation in the surface curvature. Recalling from Chapter 1 that the orientation of the joint reaction force is controlled in large part by the direction of the muscle force, we can recognize the advantage of maintaining the orientation of the patellar ligament with respect to the tib-

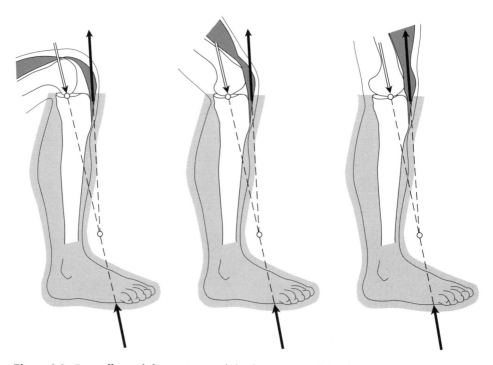

**Figure 3.3.** Regardless of the position of the knee joint, if the functional load remains constant, the orientation and point of application of the joint compressive force will not move substantially. This is because the line of application of the muscle force does not change dramatically.

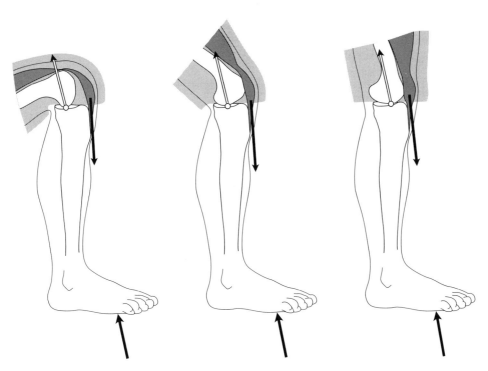

**Figure 3.4.** The joint contact force on the femur varies greatly in orientation with respect to the femur. This is due mostly to the change in orientation of the patellar ligament force with respect to the femur as the joint moves through its range of motion.

ial plateau. Notice that there is only a small variation in the direction of the patellar ligament force with respect to the tibia throughout the entire range of motion of the knee joint. In our illustration we show a constant force acting on the foot. The required joint reaction force for equilibrium varies little in its orientation relative to the tibial plateau. In each of the three positions, the joint reaction force can be produced by joint compression loading.

Let's perform a similar analysis for the femur. Joint contact forces with regard to the distal femoral condyles can endure a relatively large variation in angular orientation (Fig. 3.4). Just as we examined the orientation of the patellar ligament force with respect to the tibial plateau, we will now examine the patellar ligament force and its orientation relative to the femur. Notice that as the knee flexes, the orientation of the patellar tendon force changes markedly with respect to the femoral axis. However, observation will show that the orientation remains essentially parallel to the line that is perpendicular to the femoral condyles at its point of contact with the tibia. Thus, the large range in joint contact location on the femoral condyle is accompanied by and closely coupled with a similarly large range in orientation of muscle force in the extension mechanism.

Muscle forces have a secondary effect on joint stability. Consider the shoulder joint shown in Figure 3.5. In the abducted position, the functional

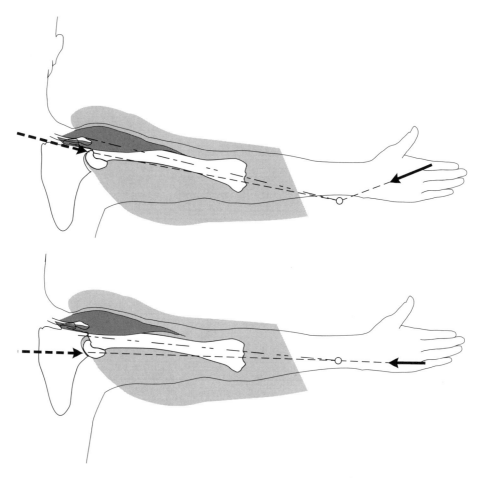

**Figure 3.5.** For the functional load shown, with the arm in abduction, joint reaction force is supplied by joint compressive load on the superior portion of the glenoid. A small change in the orientation of the functional load moves the head of the humerus inferiorly, changes the angle of orientation of the deltoid muscle with respect to the humerus, and allows joint equilibrium with a joint compressive load on the inferior margin of the glenoid.

adduction load is resisted by the contraction of the deltoid muscle. Small changes in the orientation and magnitude of the functional load cause small changes in the orientation of the joint reaction. Because the glenoid has a curvature slightly larger than that of the humerus, small amounts of humeral motion occur as the joint seeks its stable position. When the required joint reaction force on the humerus is tipped superiorly, the humerus slides inferiorly on the glenoid surface, seeking a new equilibrium position. This also has the effect of changing the orientation of the deltoid tendon force with respect to the humerus. Note that the new force differs from the muscle force required to balance the adduction load by a small amount. This small change in load applied to the humerus changes the requirement for the joint reaction force by an identical amount. This change in the required joint reaction force allows the joint contact load to provide equilibrium without having to make contact at the extreme distal, inferior border of the glenoid.

Notice that this mechanism is a coupling between two common factors of joint geometry. The first factor is that a joint must undergo relative motion to change the point of application and, hence, the direction of the joint contact force. The second factor is that the small change in relative position of joint surfaces provides meaningful changes in orientation of the resulting muscle force. Consider the example of the finger joint in Figure 3.6. When the functional load is changed, the point of contact on the joint surface moves from a superior to an inferior position. Without changing the angle of flexion, there may be correspondingly large changes in the orientation of the resulting muscle force. It is important to distinguish this statement from that previously made regarding the relatively constant direction of muscle force throughout the range of motion. These large rotations (typically 90 degrees or more) do not of themselves produce significant changes in muscle force orientation. Rather, meaningful changes in the orientation of the muscle force are caused by the motion of the condyle parallel to the contact surface while the joint seeks a stable position.

Besides the effects of joint surface geometry and muscle forces, passive ligament forces also provide a mechanism of joint stability. The role of providing joint stability while still allowing an unrestricted range of motion requires a careful balance of ligament properties and geometry. For example, consider the fact that under passive, normal joint motion, no ligament spanning a joint

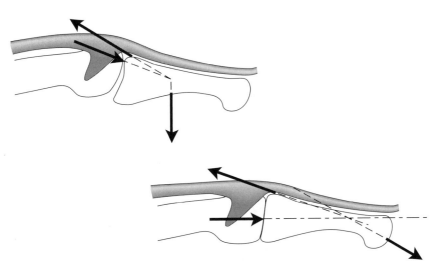

**Figure 3.6.** Large changes in functional load cause large changes in the point of contact on joint surfaces. This can result in alterations in the line of application of the muscle force.

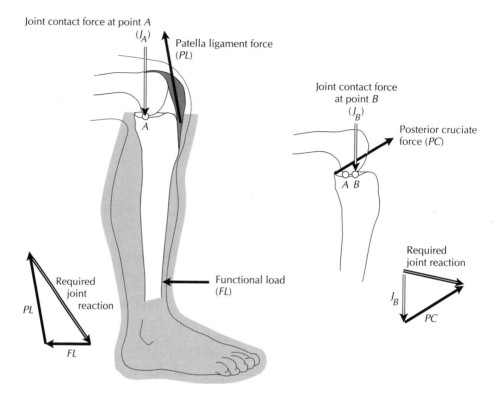

**Figure 3.7.** At the contact position shown (point *A*), the joint contact force cannot provide the required joint reaction. When the femur moves to contact at point *B*, the posterior cruciate ligament will stretch and pull anteriorly and proximally on the tibia. When these two forces ($J_B$ and *PC*) are added, they produce the required joint reaction force.

develops appreciable tensile force. Any force that a ligament produces in stabilizing the joint must be the result of subtle differences in joint motion between those motions induced under load and those motions induced passively.

Ligaments provide joint stability in the plane of motion by a mechanism that uses constraining force in the direction of motion. This mechanism is typified by the knee joint (Fig. 3.7). At the instant in time depicted, the external functional load is creating a joint reaction force that does not lie perpendicular to the tibial plateau, even if the femur made contact near the anterior rim of the plateau.

To generate the required joint reaction force, the femur slides anteriorly on the tibia, stretching the posterior cruciate ligament and thereby creating tension within the ligament. This ligament tensile force provides the missing component of the joint reaction force. Thus, the joint remains stable, since it has undergone only 2 to 3 millimeters of displacement while maintaining contact on the articular regions of its surfaces. In a similar manner, posterior motion of the femur relative to the tibia can stretch the anterior cruciate ligament.

If the joint stability provided by the mechanism of motion of the contact point along the curvature of the joint surface is to be effective, the cruciate ligaments must allow some anterior and posterior relative joint motion without producing ligament tension. This means that anteroposterior knee joint motion should be allowed in the midrange of joint surface contact without ligament tension. However, with motion in either an extreme anterior or posterior position of joint contact, ligament tension should gradually increase and effectively prevent further joint motion past the extreme point of joint surface contact. To summarize, the property of the ligament that is important in providing this first mechanism of joint stability is a "dead" zone, in which the joint is free to find a position of stability based upon joint curvature and the direction of the joint reaction. If an equilibrium position does not lie within this central range, increased excursion of the joint must induce ligament tension that will contribute directly to joint stability. Measurements of the tensile forces generated in the anterior cruciate ligament for simulated passive and active knee motion have been made on human cadaveric material (1) (Fig. 3.8). These activities would not be expected to require cruciate ligament force for joint stability. Note the large range of motion over which no anterior cruciate ligament force was detected.

It is desirable to have the stabilizing ligament forces oriented as close as possible to the direction of relative motion of the joint surfaces. Thus, if a ligament is to prevent anteroposterior motion, its orientation must be primarily in an anteroposterior direction. Further, if the tensile forces induced in the ligament are not to create moments tending to disturb the equilibrium, the ligament must pass close to the center of rotation of the joint.

The properties that we have described as desirable are found in the cruciate ligaments of the knee. To examine the properties of the anterior cruciate

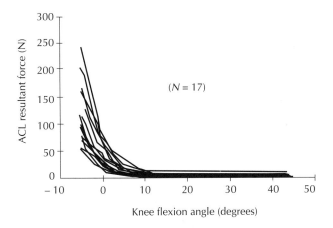

**Figure 3.8.** These curves representing cadaver cruciate ligament load versus knee position were obtained for two loading conditions. The first condition was manual extension of the lower leg against gravity, and the second was extension of the lower leg by application of a 200-newton tension on the quadriceps tendon (1).

**Figure 3.9.** The tensile load-versus-elongation curve for an anterior cruciate ligament obtained from a 22-year-old cadaver (2).

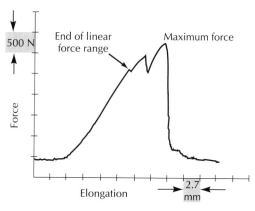

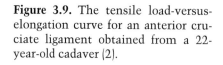

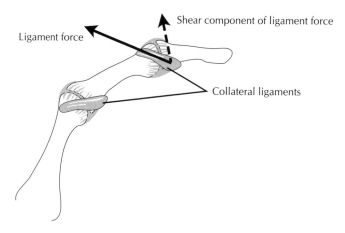

**Figure 3.10.** Finger joint showing shear forces generated by the collateral ligaments.

ligament, for example, we begin by sectioning all the structures connecting the knee joint except the anterior cruciate ligament. We can then pull apart the femur and the tibia along the direction of the remaining ligament. The mechanical behavior of the ligament can then be determined by simultaneously measuring and recording the length of the ligament and the applied force (2). A typical curve of load versus elongation is shown in Figure 3.9. Note that an excursion of approximately 5 millimeters from the initial resting position of the knee joint must be induced before even a slight increase in tension is noted in the ligament. This corresponds to the clinical observation of a lax or "loose" region in the knee joint, whereby minimal alternating anterior and posterior force can produce an excursion of up to 7 millimeters in the normal knee (3). This lax region represents the range of contact points that the joint surfaces are free to seek before engaging the ligaments to assist and stabilize the joint.

While our example has dealt with intracapsular ligaments, collateral ligaments can also function with the same mechanism. In the proximal interphalangeal joint of the hand, the collateral ligaments are relatively narrow bands of strongly oriented fibers (Fig. 3.10). When the joint reaction force must provide a large shear component (a component parallel to the articular surface), the collateral ligaments must be stretched. This induces a force that has a large component parallel to the joint surface. In this way, the collateral ligaments act much like the cruciate ligaments of the knee. Note that the collateral ligaments are capable of providing shear forces in both dorsal and volar directions. Also note the relation between the location of induced ligament force and the center of rotation of the joint.

## Mechanisms in the Lateral Plane

As we learned in Chapter 1, equilibrium requires a balance of forces in all directions. Therefore, when a medially directed force is applied to the foot during gait (Fig. 3.11), both a moment and a laterally directed force must be applied to the tibia at the knee joint. If we apply the conditions of equilibrium

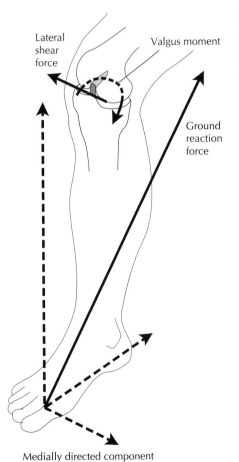

Lateral
shear
force

Valgus moment

Ground
reaction
force

Medially directed component
of ground reaction force

**Figure 3.11.** During the stance phase of gait, the femur applies both a lateral shear force and a valgus moment to the proximal tibia to balance the effect of the medial component of the ground reaction force (4).

**Figure 3.12.** A small medial shift of the tibia produces changes to the joint contact and ligament forces that tend to move the tibia laterally.

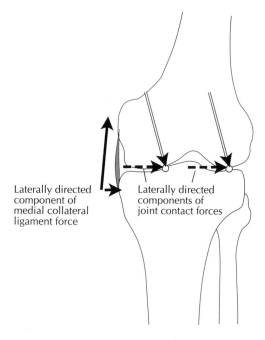

Laterally directed component of medial collateral ligament force

Laterally directed components of joint contact forces

to the tibia, we see that the laterally directed force at the knee must be equal to the medially directed component of the ground reaction force, and the valgus moment applied to the proximal tibia must be equal to the medially directed component multiplied by the length of the lower limb.

Let's first describe how the knee joint produces the laterally directed force on the tibia. When a medially directed ground reaction force is applied, it tends to move the tibia medially with respect to the femur (Fig. 3.12). This causes a small shift in the region of contact at the femorotibial articular surface. Instead of being located centrally on the lateral plateau, the contact region shifts toward the lateral side. Remembering that the joint reaction force must always be perpendicular to the joint contact surfaces, we note that the region of contact no longer has its surface parallel to the ground. Instead, the surface is tipped. Drawing a perpendicular to the surface shows that the joint reaction force would also be tipped. We can now resolve this force into two components, and we note that the horizontal component is equal in magnitude to the medially directed component of the ground reaction force. Because the knee joint surfaces have close conformity in the lateral plane, only a very small lateral displacement of the tibia is necessary to produce this shift in the contact region.

All medial shifts of joint surfaces are accompanied by a stretching of the collateral ligaments (and, in the knee joint, the cruciate ligaments as well). Stretching the ligaments induces tensile forces in the ligaments that increase the joint reaction force and, thus, its transverse component. With the joint in its displaced position, the collateral ligaments are oriented so as to produce a laterally directed component of force on the tibia. Thus, we see that the joint surfaces and the ligaments work in a coupled fashion so that the transverse forces necessary for stability can be produced by small translations of the joint surfaces.

The varus bending moment created at the knee joint by the medial component of the ground reaction force is balanced by a valgus moment created within the knee joint. The mechanisms for producing this moment, while different from those just described, nevertheless involve the joint surfaces and the ligaments. There are three mechanisms by which this valgus moment is produced in the knee joint. To understand these mechanisms, we will examine the knee joint during the stance phase of gait. The nominal ground reaction, patellar ligament, and joint reaction forces are shown (Fig. 3.13). Let's examine the contact and pressure distribution pattern of the knee joint when no varus or valgus moment is applied (Fig. 3.14). The pressure distribution results in a net contact force acting on the tibia that is in balance (equilibrium) with the patellar ligament and the ground reaction forces.

Under the influence of a varus moment, the pressure distribution within the tibiofemoral contact surfaces changes to produce increased pressure in the medial compartment of the knee and reduced pressure in the lateral com-

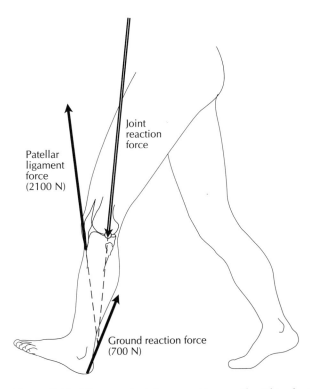

**Figure 3.13.** The nominal forces acting on the tibia during heel strike are shown.

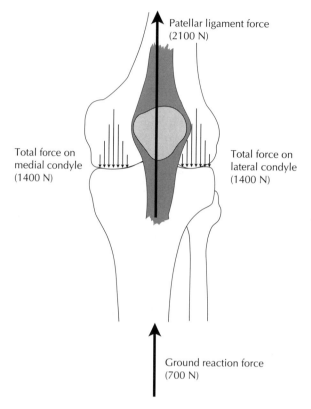

**Figure 3.14.** If the ground reaction force has no component producing either varus or valgus moments, the components of the joint contact forces on the medial and lateral condyles are equal.

partment (Fig. 3.15). We may think of this as a shifting of the location of the net contact force in the medial direction. Based upon the principle of equilibrium, the sum of the moments produced by the ground reaction force, the force in the patellar ligament, and the joint reaction force must be zero. At this point, we do not know the exact location of the net joint contact force, so let's designate its location as some distance, $x$, from the center of the patellar ligament. For this example, gait studies show us that the ground reaction force passes 0.06 meters medial to the center of the patellar ligament, or $(0.06 - x)$ meters medial to the joint contact force. We also know the magnitudes of both the ground reaction force $(F_{GR})$ and the force in the patellar ligament $(F_{PatLig})$.

We can now sum the varus and valgus moments about the unknown joint contact point:

$$[F_{PatLig} \times x \text{ m}] - [F_{GR} \times (0.06 - x) \text{ m}] = 0$$
$$[2100 \text{ N} \times x \text{ m}] - [700 \text{ N} \times (0.06 - x) \text{ m}] = 0$$

where we have adopted the convention that varus moments are positive quantities and valgus moments are negative quantities. We can use the moment equation to solve for $x$:

$$x = 0.015 \text{ m}$$

So lateral equilibrium is maintained in the knee joint during the early stance phase of normal gait by shifting the location of the net contact force 1.5 centimeters medially.

Shifting of the location of the net contact force requires an altered pressure distribution that is accomplished by a small varus rotation of the tibia about the femur. The initial loading of the joint surfaces produces cartilage deformations of about 0.2 millimeters. Relaxing the lateral deformation to 0.1 millimeters and increasing the medial deformation to 0.3 millimeters will produce the necessary change in the joint contact pressure distribution. The amount of varus angulation required to produce this change in the pattern of surface deformation is less than 1 degree.

If we examine the ground reaction force when a subject changes direction rapidly, we will find an apparently impossible result. The subject has a large medially directed component of the ground reaction force and, thus, the line of

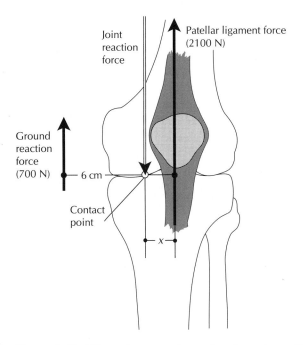

**Figure 3.15.** When the ground reaction force is applied medial to the knee joint, the joint reaction force shifts medially. Thus, the varus moment on the tibia caused by the ground reaction force is balanced by the valgus moment caused by the shift of the joint reaction force.

action of the ground reaction force vector passes the knee at a larger distance (0.15 meters) than in the example of normal gait (0.06 meters). The force in the patellar ligament does not differ from that found for normal gait (2100 newtons), because the flexion moment that must be counterbalanced by this force does not differ from the case of normal gait.

When balancing the varus and valgus moments about the joint contact point, however, we find that solving for the distance, $x$, gives rise to a contact point off the surface of the knee joint:

$$[2100 \text{ N} \times x \text{ m}] - [700 \text{ N} \times (0.15 - x) \text{ m}] = 0$$

$$x = 0.0375 \text{ m}$$

Because this tibia is only 60 millimeters (0.06 meters) wide, the "joint contact force" is not being applied to the joint surfaces, but rather 7.5 millimeters medial to the medial tibial border. Such an impossible physical finding means that we have incorrectly defined the problem. In reality, once the joint contact point reaches the most medial aspect of the joint surface, further varus moment production can be generated only by increasing the magnitude of the joint contact force or allowing the joint to undergo further varus angulation until the lateral collateral ligament stretches.

Increasing the magnitude of the joint contact force is the second mechanism, therefore, for providing joint stability in the lateral plane in response to varus or valgus loading. This mechanism also requires a bicondylar joint that can shift the contact regions between the medial and lateral condyles. The moment is still produced by the eccentric joint load, but the joint load is not simply the equilibrium response of the functional load and the muscle force. When this second mechanism is used, the joint reaction force is augmented in such a way that the net moment in the plane of motion (flexion-extension) is not changed, but the joint contact force is increased.

In our current example, equilibrium of the lower leg at this phase of the gait cycle requires a 105-newton-meter extension moment to be applied to the tibia at the knee joint. This moment can be produced by 2100 newtons of tension applied through the patellar ligament (Fig. 3.13). We may also voluntarily increase the force in the quadriceps muscle, creating an additional extension moment, and balance this unnecessary additional extension moment by a moment created by tensing the hamstring muscles. Let's assume that an additional 500 newtons of force is developed in the quadriceps muscle (Fig. 3.16). The moment arm of the hamstring muscles is 0.07 meters, as compared with the moment arm for the patellar ligament, which is 0.05 meters. We can calculate the force in the hamstring muscles ($F_{Ham}$) necessary to maintain a 105-newton-meter extension moment by considering moment equilibrium (Equation 1.4):

$$105 \text{ N} \cdot \text{m} - (F_{PatLig} \times 0.05 \text{ m}) + (F_{Ham} \times 0.07 \text{ m}) = 0$$

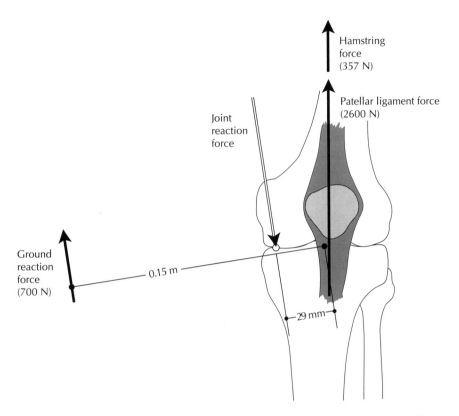

**Figure 3.16.** When the ground reaction force is shifted 0.15 meters medially during a quick turn, the joint reaction force can be maintained on the medial condyle by augmenting the patellar ligament force and contracting the hamstring muscles.

Substituting for the patellar ligament force (2100 newtons plus the additional 500 newtons),

$$105 \text{ N} \cdot \text{m} - (2600 \text{ N} \times 0.05 \text{ m}) + (F_{\text{Ham}} \times 0.07 \text{ m}) = 0$$

Solving for the force in the hamstring muscles yields

$$F_{\text{Ham}} = \frac{2600 \text{ N} \times 0.05 \text{ m} - 105 \text{ N} \cdot \text{m}}{0.07 \text{ m}}$$

$$= 357 \text{ N}$$

We must now reconsider equilibrium of the varus and valgus moments about the joint contact point (Fig. 3.16):

$$(2600 \text{ N} \times x) + (357 \text{ N} \times x) - [700 \text{ N} \times (0.15 \text{ m} - x)] = 0$$

Solving for x yields

$$x = 0.029 \text{ m}$$

Thus, by augmenting both the agonist and antagonist muscle forces, we can maintain joint stability by allowing the contact point of the joint compressive force to shift 29 millimeters toward the medial side of the medial condyle. In doing this, however, we pay a penalty in terms of the magnitude of the joint compressive load. By increasing the quadriceps force and adding a hamstrings force, we increase the joint compressive force required to maintain equilibrium. In addition, we are loading the medial edge of the medial condyle.

The joint compressive force magnitude is approximately equal to the vertical component of the ground reaction force, plus the tension in both the quadriceps and hamstring muscles. Thus, the joint reaction force is increased by 31 percent, from approximately 2800 newtons to 3657 newtons. In addition, the joint angulation will be increased to about 1 degree because of the increased compressive load on the medial compartment. By shifting the joint load to the medial compartment (because of the primary mechanism for joint stability) and by augmenting the joint load (by the second mechanism for stability), we have increased the medial joint compartment load from about one-half the initial joint reaction (1400 newtons) to over two and one-half times that value. For a 700-newton-weight individual, this is a medial compartment load of over five times body weight.

This mechanism of augmenting the joint compressive load can be appreciated by examining the proximal interphalangeal (PIP) joint of the index finger during the function of key pinch (Fig. 3.17). In this function, there is no flexion or extension moment applied to the PIP joint. The functional load is a force in the ulnar direction on the distal phalange. To stabilize the PIP joint, tension is developed in both the flexor and extensor tendon groups. This creates sufficient joint compressive load to allow equilibrium to be achieved by establishing joint contact on the medial condyle.

There are situations in which the method of load augmentation is either unavailable or insufficient to maintain joint stability. The mechanism may be unavailable if the force producing angulation of the joint is applied unexpectedly and rapidly. Contraction of both agonist and antagonist muscle groups requires a certain amount of reaction time, which might not be available in some circumstances. The augmentation mechanism might be insufficient if the magnitude of the muscle force required to resist flexion or extension is at or near a maximal contraction level. For example, a weakened individual performing normal activities or a well-trained athlete performing a maximal activity may not have the reserve muscle strength required for this augmentation mechanism. In these cases, varus or valgus moments of large magnitude will result first in the shifting of the center of pressure of the joint contact force to an extreme position, followed by separation of the articulating surfaces between the unloaded condyles.

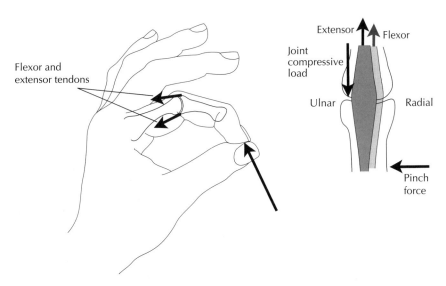

**Figure 3.17.** When pinch force is applied to the distal phalanx of the first finger, the proximal interphalangeal joint is stabilized by a joint compressive force. The joint compressive force is created by concurrent action of the flexion and extension mechanisms. The joint reaction force is centered on the ulnar side of the joint, creating the needed valgus moment to counterbalance the varus moment created by the pinch force.

If, in the example presented in Figure 3.16, we are dealing with an individual without sufficient muscle strength to augment the muscle forces, what ligamentous loading will be induced? Let's assume that the separation of the medial joint surfaces will produce tension in only the lateral collateral ligament. We will ignore the cruciate ligaments and will support this assumption later. For the joint configuration shown in Figure 3.18, moment equilibrium of the lower leg requires that the sum of the moments about the center of the joint reaction force in the medial compartment equal zero. This contact point has assumed a medial position, giving a moment arm for the tension developed in the lateral collateral ligament of 0.075 meters. To find the tension in the ligament, we apply the principle of moment equilibrium (Equation 1.4) to sum the moments due to the ground reaction force $(F_{GR})$, the patellar ligament force $(F_{PatLig})$, and the lateral collateral ligament force $(F_{LCL})$ and set the sum equal to zero:

$$(F_{GR} \times 0.13 \text{ m}) - (F_{PatLig} \times 0.020 \text{ m}) - (F_{LCL} \times 0.055 \text{ m}) = 0$$

Substituting the values for the ground reaction force (700 newtons) and the patellar ligament force (2100 newtons), we can solve for the force in the lateral collateral ligament:

$$(700 \text{ N} \times 0.13 \text{ m}) - (2100 \text{ N} \times 0.020 \text{ m}) - (F_{LCL} \times 0.055 \text{ m}) = 0$$

$$F_{LCL} = 891 \text{ N}$$

While this load is large compared with the strength of cadaver ligaments (5), it is probably a maximally acceptable load for a young, healthy ligament.

We can now calculate the joint compressive load. It is approximately equal to the sum of the vertical component of the ground reaction force, the force in the patellar ligament, and the force in the lateral collateral ligament. This results in a joint compressive load of 3691 newtons. This is an increase in joint reaction force of 891 newtons as compared with the joint reaction force occurring when only the primary mechanism of joint stability is active. It is about the same as the increase required by the joint stability mechanism of load augmentation. The required 891 newtons of tension in the medial collateral ligament can be produced only by stretching the ligament. Since the elongation for the collateral ligament near its maximum load is approximately 20 percent (5), the 25-millimeter-long ligament will elongate 5 millimeters. This elongation of the medial collateral ligament corresponds to a varus angulation of 5 degrees.

We can now examine our assumption that separation of the joint surfaces produces tension primarily in the lateral collateral ligament. To do this,

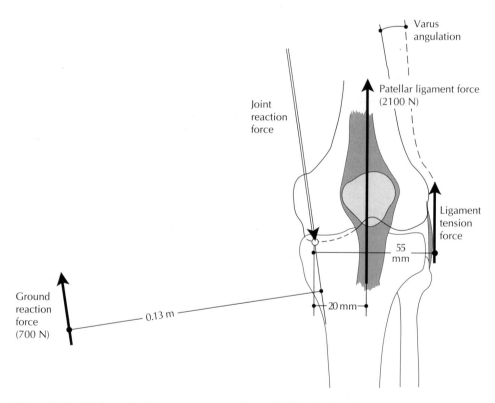

**Figure 3.18.** Without load augmentation, the medially displaced ground reaction force will require lateral collateral ligament tension to keep the tibia in equilibrium. For the loads shown, the tibia will rotate into 5 degrees of varus.

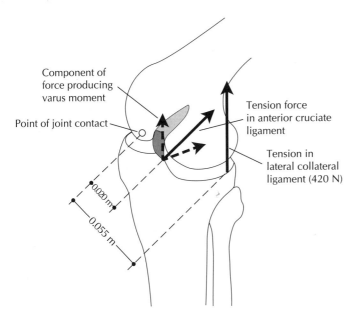

Component of
force producing
varus moment

Point of joint contact

Tension force
in anterior cruciate
ligament

Tension in
lateral collateral
ligament (420 N)

0.020 m

0.055 m

**Figure 3.19.** Only a small component of the force in the anterior cruciate ligament acts vertically so as to generate a valgus moment on the tibia. Its moment arm is only 0.02 meters, much shorter than the moment arm enjoyed by the lateral collateral ligament.

we will determine the contribution of the anterior cruciate ligament to the varus stability of the knee in this situation. We observe in Figure 3.19 that the anterior cruciate ligament is not aligned vertically and, therefore, only a component of its tension (approximately one-half) will contribute to producing a valgus moment. Since the anterior cruciate ligament's origin and insertion are closer to the center of the joint contact area than are those of the lateral collateral ligament, the varus angulation of the lower leg will stretch the anterior cruciate ligament proportionately less. In this case, the elongation is only about 30 percent of that experienced by the lateral collateral ligament due both to its closer location to the joint contact point and its oblique orientation. Examining Figure 3.9, we see that this induces about 400 newtons of tensile force in the anterior cruciate ligament. Additionally, the moment arm that this force enjoys in producing a valgus moment about the joint contact point is 0.020 meters, only 36 percent of the moment arm of the lateral collateral ligament. The 400-newton anterior cruciate ligament tensile force is applied obliquely to the tibia and therefore has only a 285-newton component acting perpendicular to the tibia to produce a valgus moment. The small tensile force combined with a smaller moment arm produces only

$$M_{ACL} = 285 \text{ N} \times 0.02 \text{ m}$$

$$= 5.7 \text{ N} \cdot \text{m}$$

This moment is less than one-eighth of the valgus moment produced by the lateral collateral ligament:

$$M_{LCL} = 891 \text{ N} \times 0.055 \text{ m}$$
$$= 49.0 \text{ N} \cdot \text{m}$$

We have now considered three mechanisms by which planar joints such as the knee generate resisting moments in directions perpendicular to the primary plane of motion. The first mechanism involves shifting the joint contact point so as to produce a moment by action of the same force that provides equilibrium in the plane of motion. In our example of the knee, the patellar ligament force provides this double duty, by creating both extension and valgus moments about the shifted joint contact point. Only a certain maximum moment arm can be created by this mechanism, however, because while the magnitude of the force is determined by the activity, the maximum amount of shift in the joint contact point is limited by the size and shape of the joint.

If the required valgus moment exceeds the capacity of this mechanism, there are two alternatives. The quadriceps muscle can produce a stronger contractile force, though this will necessitate a similar increase in the force in the hamstring muscles, so as to maintain an appropriate extension moment to balance the flexion moment created by the ground reaction force. When the joint contact point shifts medially, the increased forces in the patellar ligament and in the hamstring muscles both contribute to a larger valgus moment to balance the varus moment generated by the ground reaction force. This mechanism does not require opening of the lateral joint compartment, only shifting of the joint contact point; therefore, no force is produced in the lateral collateral ligament.

The third mechanism for obtaining varus-valgus joint equilibrium involves the opening of a joint compartment corresponding with a shift of the joint contact point to the opposite side of the joint. In our example, the opening of the joint allowed the lateral collateral ligament to be stretched, creating a tensile ligamentous force. The moment created by this force about the medially located joint contact point maintains the varus-valgus moment equilibrium.

## STABILITY IN NORMAL AND ABNORMAL JOINTS

We have seen how joint stability depends upon the interactions of joint surfaces, muscles, and ligamentous structures. In describing mechanisms of joint stability, we have used several terms to describe relative motion. We have used the term *displacement* to mean the change in position of one bone with respect to another. *We have considered displacement as consisting of two components: translation and rotation. Translation is relative motion where all points on a moving object travel in parallel paths.* Thus, if a vertically oriented tibia translates to a new position, the tibia will still be vertical. *Rotation is relative motion where all points on a moving object travel in circular paths about a point that may or may not be within the object.* We have also used the term *angulation* with the same definition.

In evaluating joint stability in the plane of motion, we recognize the importance of the anteroposterior position of the joint contact point in initiating the mechanisms dependent upon joint curvature, muscle force, and ligamentous restraint. Furthermore, the relative anteroposterior position of the joint under functional load enters into our definition of joint stability. We therefore define *joint laxity for motion in the flexion-extension plane as the total anteroposterior translation that can be produced within the joint by the application of an arbitrarily chosen, fixed-amplitude force alternating between the anterior and posterior directions.*

The conditions under which the joint is tested for laxity will vary depending upon the clinical question. The joint is tested in an unloaded condition (with neither functional load nor muscle force applied to the limb) if only the ligamentous contribution to joint stability is to be detected. In many cases, however, examining unloaded joints will not completely eliminate the contribution to stability provided by the curvature of the joint surfaces. This is especially true if the tensile forces induced in the ligaments crossing the joint create a joint contact force. Obviously, tests that allow or induce joint contact forces cannot separate the stability contribution of the ligaments from that of the joint surface curvatures. Therefore, while our definition of joint laxity applies to all conditions of testing, the resultant laxity is dependent not only on the chosen amplitude of the anteroposterior load, but on all other test conditions as well.

The definition of joint laxity also applies to the measurements in the lateral plane. Here we use two measurements, translational laxity and rotational laxity. *Translational laxity is the medial-lateral translation induced by an alternating medial-lateral load of arbitrarily chosen amplitude.* All the conditions and couplings appropriate to anteroposterior translational laxity apply to medial-lateral translational laxity. *Rotational laxity is the change in varus or valgus angle produced by an alternating varus or valgus moment of arbitrarily chosen amplitude.* The conditions of joint loading, such as muscle tension or angle of flexion, will obviously affect both laxity measurements in the lateral plane.

Associated with the concept of joint laxity is the term *neutral position*. It is convenient to separate the structures of a joint providing anterior stability from those structures providing posterior stability. Unfortunately, anterior and posterior stability are seldom provided by separate, identifiable structures. But such a classification is often appealing. If the anteroposterior displacement in the plane of motion is to be separated into an anterior component and a posterior component, then some point of demarcation, termed a *neutral position*, must be chosen. *A neutral position may be arbitrarily defined for any test system as the position assumed by the joint when there is neither anterior nor posterior applied load.* Although this is a reasonable and concise definition, it does not distinguish a unique relative position of the joint surfaces. As an example, in the knee joint with an absent anterior cruciate ligament, the joint may find an unloaded resting point over a range of several millimeters of

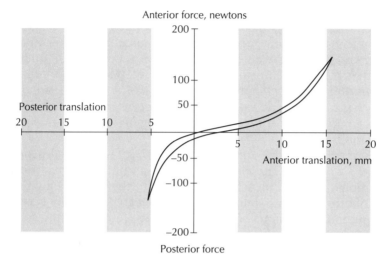

**Figure 3.20.** With an absent anterior cruciate ligament, the "dead zone" of the knee flexed 30 degrees is approximately 5 millimeters in length. Application of a small joint compressive load could bring the joint to rest anywhere along this zone (6).

anteroposterior displacement (Fig. 3.20). Furthermore, the application of a joint compressive load will produce a joint excursion and, hence, a different resting or neutral position. In general, the neutral position is highly dependent upon joint configuration, the integrity of the connecting soft tissues, and the intensity of the joint compressive load.

## STABILITY IN JOINTS WITH LIGAMENTOUS INJURIES

We recognize that ligamentous constraint is an important, though not a primary, mechanism of joint stability. We have seen how joint curvature in combination with joint compressive load and muscle force can constitute the primary stabilizing mechanisms. However, the most common injuries affecting joint mechanics are injuries to ligamentous structures. The mechanism is straightforward. The ligaments are the secondary system evoked when applied forces exceed the capability of the primary system. This ordering or sequential utilization of stability mechanisms gives rise to problems in the diagnosis of joint injury. The function of the secondary ligamentous system can be examined in isolation only if the primary system is somehow excluded. In many instances, this is either impractical or impossible. To further complicate the issue, all major joints have redundant ligamentous structures.

To understand the mechanics of the behavior of a joint with a ligamentous injury, let's first look at the mechanical behavior of the injured ligament itself. The load-versus-elongation curve for the anterior cruciate ligament (Fig. 3.9) portrays the behavior in its normal or reversible operating range, as well as its behavior in the damaged range. After the initial reversible range, discontinuities are noted in the curve. Each of these small discontinuities represents failure in isolated fibers or fiber bundles. During the initial flat portion of the loading curve, fibers were straightened and then sequentially recruited to bear load. A similar sequencing takes place in the failure region. Fibers reach their ultimate strength and then rupture, sequentially dumping load on the remaining fibers.

If the loading mechanism on the joint produces a controlled, excessive elongation, such as might occur in a rugby pileup, failure may be limited to the rupture of some fraction of the total fiber content of the ligament. This can be seen from the load-versus-elongation curve for the anterior cruciate ligament, where the initial fiber failure occurs at approximately 70 percent of the maximum elongation.

The problem of orthopaedic diagnosis is complicated by the specific limited goals of the diagnostic procedures. We are attempting to identify the deficiency in stability. We usually employ the concepts of joint laxity and neutral position in our diagnosis. Changes in joint laxity are usually assumed to be indicative of ligamentous damage. Changes in neutral position are not as easily identified and often confuse the measurement of joint laxity.

As we have seen, ligaments may be damaged or "sprained" and still retain a considerable fraction of both their stiffness and strength. Trying to detect the difference in ligament stiffness that accompanies rupture of 10 percent of the fibers in the ligament is probably impossible in a clinical setting. Since most clinical evaluations cannot apply loads near the maximum strength of the ligament, it is unlikely that the change in stiffness of the ligament will be detectable, unless the vast majority of the fibers are ruptured.

Laboratory tests, unlike clinical evaluations, are performed either with the ligamentous structures intact or with these structures selectively sectioned. Most laboratory tests attempt to recreate clinical evaluations. We shall first examine the laboratory analog of an anterior drawer test of the knee. Depending upon the angle of knee flexion, there are three primary structures that contribute to ligamentous stability of the knee in the anteroposterior direction. In the laboratory test, unlike in the clinical analog, muscle force and, hence, joint compressive loading are inherently absent. Keeping in mind this major difference between the two situations, let's investigate the mechanics of the anterior drawer test.

The usual goal of the drawer test is to evaluate the integrity of the anterior cruciate ligament. However, the collateral ligaments also provide restraint in the anteroposterior direction. If the knee is subjected to a predetermined load in the laboratory test, say 100 newtons, the tibia will translate anteriorly with respect to the femur and, depending upon the point of application of the load, may also display some amount of axial rotation. The amount of anterior translation of the tibia depends upon the original neutral position and the final position of the tibia under load. The application of posterior force on the tibia similarly produces posterior translation and axial rotation. We see that there is a small region in the center of the load-versus-translation curve for the knee that is relatively flat (Fig. 3.21). In this region, the position of the knee is extremely sensitive to the imposed load.

If we now section the anterior cruciate ligament and repeat the laboratory test, we will find that the curve corresponding to anterior translation is altered. Therefore, it is easy to conclude that sectioning the anterior cruciate ligament allows an increased anterior translation at the 100-newton load level of approximately 9 millimeters, or an increase of approximately 180 percent. This statement can be made in confidence, since there is no change in the posterior translation characteristics of the knee when we section the anterior cruciate ligament and because we can make the comparison based upon equivalent neutral positions of the knee.

Now let's examine two situations that can complicate the formulation of conclusions regarding this laboratory test. The first situation involves a knee with intact anterior and posterior cruciate ligaments, but whose load-versus-translation behavior differs from the previous knee (Fig. 3.22). In this case, we have not defined the neutral position as of yet, but we note that the central portion of the curve has a much larger flat region, so much so that it resembles the curve we obtained after sectioning the anterior cruciate ligament in our prior laboratory test (Fig. 3.20). Determining the anterior translation is again dependent upon the choice of neutral position.

Let's assume that the mechanism for determining the neutral position consists of applying a posteriorly directed force of 5 newtons. This force tightens the posterior cruciate ligament, and we now attribute all anterior translation to

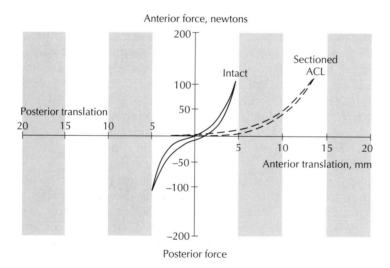

**Figure 3.21.** With or without the anterior cruciate ligament, the posterior translation of the tibia remains the same. When the anterior cruciate ligament is sectioned, anterior translation at 100 newtons of anteriorly applied force (anterior laxity) increases almost threefold (6).

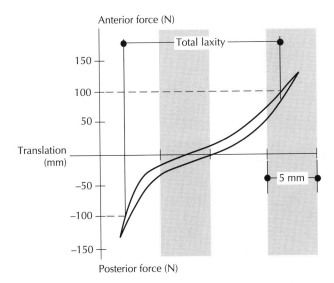

**Figure 3.22.** A normal knee may present with a large translation measured between 100 newtons posterior force and 100 newtons anterior force (total laxity).

be referenced from this position. Our previous example (Fig. 3.21) would show 5 millimeters of anterior translation under 100 newtons of load, whereas our present example (Fig. 3.23) will show 10 millimeters of anterior translation. One might come to the erroneous conclusion that the anterior cruciate ligament is absent in this knee, simply based upon the large anterior translation as measured from our defined neutral position. If we continue this experiment, by sectioning the anterior cruciate ligament, we see that the added translation at 100 newtons of force is 4 millimeters. But this represents only a 40 percent increase in total anterior translation from the neutral position. Variations of this amount of laxity between right and left knees are commonly found in the clinical population and present difficulties in prescribing absolute standards for diagnostic tests (7).

The second situation that will be examined in our laboratory evaluation is the knee with an absent posterior cruciate ligament. The load-versus-translation behavior of such a knee when subjected to anterior and posterior forces is shown in Figure 3.24. True to our expectation, the curves exhibit an elongated, flat central region. In order to measure anterior translation, we must again define a neutral position. Because of our knowledge that the posterior cruciate ligament is absent, we might logically choose the neutral position by applying some minimal, 5-newton load in the anterior direction; we could then measure our anterior translation from this neutral position. Although such a choice may be logical for this test, it complicates the comparison of the performance of this knee with the two knees we previously examined. Notice that other definitions of neutral position, such as the point on the load-versus-translation curve where the curve crosses the zero load axis, the point on the

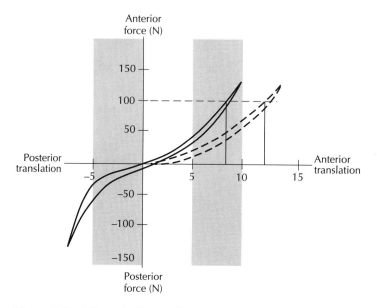

**Figure 3.23.** When the knee of Figure 3.22 suffers an anterior cruciate ligament rupture, the anterior translation of the tibia, when subjected to a 100-newton anterior load, will increase 40 percent. Contrast this with Figure 3.21, where anterior cruciate section produced a 180 percent increase in anterior translation.

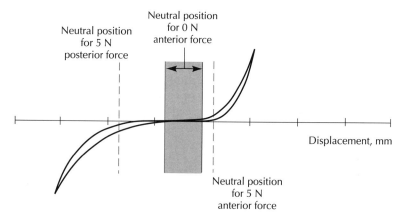

**Figure 3.24.** After sectioning of the posterior cruciate ligament, the load-translation curve of the tibia has a flat central region. If we define the neutral position by the amount of anteriorly or posteriorly applied load, we can dramatically alter the "neutral" position.

curve where the posteriorly directed force is 5 newtons, or even the midpoint on the curve between the locations of the anterior and posterior 5-newton force positions, lead to different arbitrary locations of the neutral position. Another, perhaps more appropriate method for locating the neutral position is to determine the position of the joint at rest for a particular joint compressive load for the situation in which ligamentous forces are not required for joint stability. Many variations on this theme are available in the literature (8).

The load-versus-translation curves we have examined depict whole-joint behavior. At each displacement point, several structures are resisting the applied load. Absence or alteration of any of these structures will result in changes to a portion of the curve (for example, extension of the flat central portion) or alteration of the whole curve (for example, a change in slope at every point). Applying fixed loads to a joint while measuring the joint displacements is a test usually performed in conjunction with selective ligamentous cuttings for the purpose of determining the contribution of individual ligaments to the restraint in motion. We can only answer the question, How much more will the joint move when I apply $X$ newtons of load if I remove this selected ligament? Be aware that the answer depends totally upon the condition of all other ligaments supporting that load, as well as any induced joint contact force.

Another question that is often asked is, What fraction of the applied load is resisted by a specific ligament? To answer this question requires a different test. To determine the fraction of total load carried by a particular ligament, we must construct a test in which each ligament carries a specific, reproducible load. Then we remove one ligament and, while keeping the load constant in all the other ligaments, remeasure the total applied load. Such a test is called a constant displacement test. In this test, an intact joint is placed into an apparatus that is capable of moving the joint from its neutral position to a desired loaded position. For example, the device will take a knee joint from a neutral position to a position of 10 degrees of valgus angulation. At that position, the device measures the applied valgus moment. When the moment at 10 degrees of angulation has been recorded, the knee is returned to the neutral position, and the anterior cruciate ligament is sectioned. The knee is then returned to the position of 10 degrees of valgus angulation, and the moment induced in the knee at this position is again recorded. The moment measured with the anterior cruciate ligament sectioned is less than that required to bring the knee to that position with an intact anterior cruciate ligament. The difference in moments represents the contribution of the anterior cruciate ligament in providing a moment to resist 10 degrees of valgus angulation.

Note that for each of the two tests, the elongation of the posterior cruciate ligament and that of the medial collateral ligament are identical since the angulation is identical. Because the elongations of these ligaments are the same in both tests, their induced loads are the same. Thus, the only change in the total loading of the structures supporting the knee joint is due to the absence of the anterior cruciate ligament. Therefore, we can determine the loading contribution of the anterior cruciate ligament by simple subtraction.

The experiment can be repeated by returning the knee to the neutral position and sectioning the posterior cruciate ligament. Displacement of the knee to the position of 10 degrees of valgus angulation will induce a new, even lower total moment, and subtraction of this moment from that produced in the presence of the posterior cruciate ligament will give the contribution of the posterior cruciate ligament. With both the anterior and posterior cruciate ligaments absent, the recorded moment at 10 degrees of valgus angulation is the contribution of the medial collateral ligament (assuming the absence of other supporting structures).

This experiment will work regardless of the order in which the ligaments are sectioned. The contribution of each ligament to the load-carrying capacity of a joint cannot be determined by applying a load up to some maximum (for example, 100 newtons). In this case, sectioning a ligament will not change the induced load of 100 newtons, but rather will redistribute the load among the remaining ligaments. There is no way to use this constant-load experimental method to determine the load contribution of individual elements.

If the goal of the experiment is to determine load sharing, it is important to control the mechanics of joint stability that are being examined. Remember that if a joint compressive load is added to the experiment, it must be considered as a separate, independent entity in the same way that we consider each ligament as a separate, independent entity. The entity of joint stabilization by joint compressive load has an associated load-versus-displacement characteristic for the whole joint in exactly the same way that an individual ligament has a load-versus-displacement characteristic for the whole joint.

Again, in an analogous manner, if we wish to determine the contribution of joint compressive load to the motion restraint of the joint, we may apply a constant load to the joint in the presence and then in the absence of joint compressive load. The difference in displacement of the joint can then be measured. Each magnitude and location of joint compressive load can reasonably be expected to produce a different amount of restraint under the application of anterior load (for example, 100 newtons) to the tibia. If we apply 500 newtons of joint compressive load, we would not expect to observe twice as much anterior translation of the knee under 100 newtons of anterior force as we observe when we provide 1000 newtons of joint compressive load and retest the knee with a 100-newton anterior tibial load. This is because the behavior of the knee joint contact curvatures is nonlinear. We must therefore be careful to specify *all* testing conditions, especially those involving joint compressive loads (8).

## References

1. Markolf KL, Gorek JF, Kabo JM, Shapiro MS. Direct measurement of resultant forces in the anterior cruciate ligament: an in vitro study performed with a new experimental technique. J Bone Joint Surg 1990;72A:557-567.

2. Noyes FR, Grood ES. The strength of the anterior cruciate ligament in humans and rhesus monkeys: age-related and species-related changes. J Bone Joint Surg 1976;58A:1074-1082.

3. Markolf KL, Amstutz HC. The clinical relevance of instrumented testing for ACL insufficiency. Clin Orthop 1987;223:198-207.

4. Burstein AH. Biomechanics of the knee joint. In: Insall JN, ed. Surgery of the knee. New York: Churchill Livingstone, 1984:21-39.

5. Kennedy JC, Hawkins RJ, Willis RB, and Darrylchuk KD. Tension studies of human knee ligaments: yield point, ultimate failure, and disruption of the cruciate and tibial collateral ligaments. J Bone Joint Surg 1976;58A:350-355.

6. Fukubayashi T, Torzilli PA, Sherman MF, Warren RF. An in vitro biomechanical evaluation of anterior-posterior motion of the knee: tibial displacement, rotation, and torque. J Bone Joint Surg 1982;64A:258-264.

7. Torzilli PA, Greenberg RL, Insall JN. An in vivo biomechanical evaluation of anterior-posterior motion of the knee. J Bone Joint Surg 1981;63A:960-968.

8. Markolf KL, Bargar WL, Shoemaker SC, Amstutz HC. The role of joint load in knee stability. J Bone Joint Surg 1981;63A:570-585.

# 4

## Mechanical Behavior of Materials

**STRESS**
**STRAIN**
**MODULUS OF ELASTICITY**
**MODULUS OF RIGIDITY**
**POISSON'S EFFECT**
**RELATION BETWEEN THE ELASTIC PROPERTIES**
**STRAIN ENERGY**
**STATIC LOAD BEHAVIOR**
**HYSTERESIS**
**VISCOELASTICITY**
**FAILURE CRITERIA**
**CYCLIC LOAD BEHAVIOR**

A problem that appears again and again in orthopaedic biomechanics is the prediction of the performance of biological and artificial mechanical structures. When using internal fixation to enhance fracture healing, for example, the orthopaedic surgeon must be able to predict the limits of performance of both the fracture fixation device and the damaged bone. In choosing from available total-joint-replacement implants, the surgeon must select a device with a sufficiently long functional life expectancy to meet the needs of the patient.

All predictions of the mechanical performance of any structure, be it biological or fabricated, depend on knowing the forces to which the structure will be subjected, the burdens to be placed on the materials that compose the structure, and the extent to which the material is capable of sustaining those burdens over the expected life of the structure. In our first three chapters we examined the forces exerted on structures within the musculoskeletal system while the structures performed functional tasks. In this chapter we will examine the ability of materials to withstand the mechanical burdens imposed by structures bearing these types of loads. The investigation of how loads on structures are transformed into the burdens to be carried by the materials from which the structure is fabricated will take place in Chapter 5.

## STRESS

In Chapter 1 we examined structures that were in equilibrium. We studied the loads acting on a structure by isolating the structure or a portion of the structure as a free body and applying the laws of equilibrium. This enabled us to determine the forces and moments acting across the imaginary boundary of the free body. You will remember that the boundary was chosen so that the forces and moments under question passed across the boundary. Creating an appropriate free body often required passing the boundary through a solid structure, such as a muscle, tendon, or ligament. We could just as well have passed the boundary of the free body through a bone. This would have allowed us to determine the forces and moments acting within the bone.

We must now devise a method for examining the burden placed on the material that composes a load-bearing structure. For example, while a person ambulates, what are the burdens placed upon a small piece of bone tissue located on the lateral surface of the diaphysis of the tibia? The method used to answer this question will entail the creation of a free body whose boundary coincides with a surface of the small piece of bone tissue (Fig. 4.1). We can imagine that the surface of the tibia, in order to be in equilibrium, will be subjected to some combination of loads consisting of forces and moments. Since the cortical bone tissue on this imaginary boundary is somewhat continuous (we will ignore the microscopic voids in the tissue) and somewhat homogeneous (we will also ignore the variation in density and composition due to the haversian structures in the tissue), we can assume that the loads acting on the surface are distributed in some continuous manner over the surface.

Consider the small piece of bone tissue. We might expect the surface of this piece of bone on the boundary to have forces at the "exposed" surface. If this

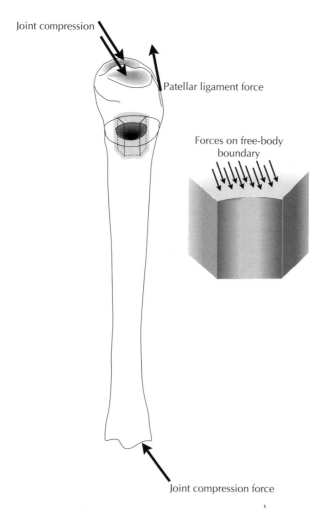

Joint compression

Patellar ligament force

Forces on free-body
boundary

Joint compression force

**Figure 4.1.** The boundary of a free body passes through the tibia. The forces and moments applied across the boundary to maintain equilibrium of the tibia result in a distribution of forces on the surface of a small piece of bone tissue.

piece of bone is small enough, we can ignore any variation of forces applied to its upper surface and consider this minute area of bone to have a uniformly distributed force across its surface. We will define the term *stress* as the condition of load existing on this minute upper surface of the piece of bone tissue in the lateral cortex of the tibia.

In general terms, *stress is a uniformly distributed force acting on a particular small surface of a defined block of material.* The intensity of the stress is calculated by the magnitude of the force divided by the amount of surface area over which the force acts:

$$\text{Stress} = \frac{\text{Force}}{\text{Area}} \qquad (4.1)$$

The units of stress are newtons/meter$^2$. In the international system of units, 1 newton/meter$^2$ is called a pascal (1 Pa).

In our example, the direction of the force acting on the small piece of tibial bone is positioned obliquely with respect to the surface of the piece. In such a case, we commonly resolve the force into two components, one acting perpendicular and one acting parallel to the surface (Fig. 4.2). We further refine our definition of stress by calling *normal stress the condition produced by the component of force acting perpendicular ($F_\perp$) to the surface* and *shear stress the condition produced by the component of force acting parallel ($F_\parallel$) to the surface:*

$$\text{Normal stress} = \frac{F_\perp}{\text{Area}}$$

(4.2)

$$\text{Shear stress} = \frac{F_\parallel}{\text{Area}}$$

Notice that our definition of stress serves as a convenient analytical tool to solve problems of equilibrium, since it relates the stresses acting on the boundaries of free bodies to the forces and the areas. However, the definition does not allow easy physical measurement. We can imagine cutting the surface of the tibia with our free-body boundary and calculating the forces it must bear, but we cannot attach a measurement gauge to that surface without actually cutting the bone and thus destroying the system. The exception to our inability to directly measure stress occurs in fluid systems (systems composed of gases and liquids). In these systems, we can measure the normal stress (usually called

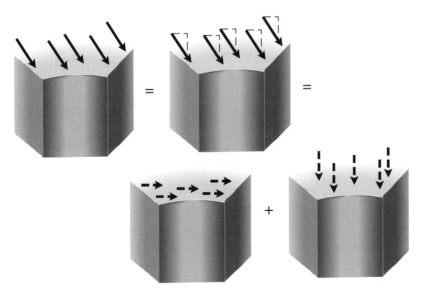

**Figure 4.2.** The oblique forces distributed on the surface of the piece of bone can be resolved into force components parallel and perpendicular to the surface.

the fluid pressure or hydrostatic pressure) simply by immersing a pressure gauge at the desired location. Typical pressures in fluids are atmospheric pressure, equal to approximately 100,000 pascals or 0.1 megapascals (MPa), where the prefix "mega" means one million, and normal diastolic blood pressure, equal to about 80 millimeters of mercury, corresponding to about 10,600 pascals. Note that 1 pascal is a very low-intensity pressure, equal to only about seven-thousandths of a millimeter of mercury.

## Normal Stress

Let's apply the definition of stress to the problem of finding the burden placed on the fibers of a muscle tendon (Fig. 4.3). To create the extension moment needed for equilibrium at the wrist joint, the muscle must produce a 50-newton contractile force. This tensile force must be transported through the tendon. To determine the stress (the intensity of the load) in the tendon, we will analyze a small portion of the tendon as a free body (Fig. 4.3). Note that in isolating the free body, we have imagined cuts through the muscle belly and through the tendon.

We have established that the force across the muscle belly must have a magnitude of 50 newtons. What is the stress on the transverse surface of the tendon? The principle of force equilibrium (Equation 1.3) applied to the free

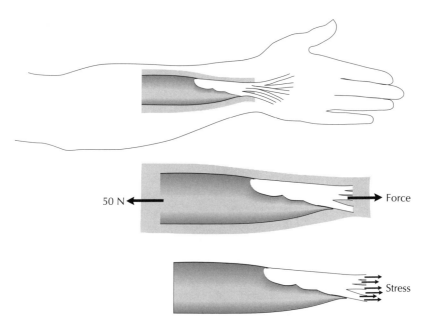

**Figure 4.3.** A muscle providing an extension moment at the wrist joint produces a contractile force of 50 newtons. Equilibrium of the free body consisting of a portion of the muscle belly and its adjoining tendon requires a 50-newton force in the tendon.

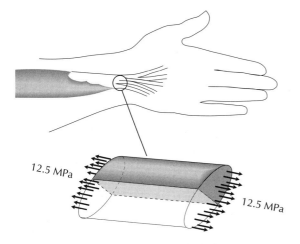

**Figure 4.4.** The stress on the longitudinal surface of the portion of the tendon from Figure 4.3 is zero.

body of the segment of muscle and tendon requires that the sum of the forces in the direction parallel to the long axis of the muscle and tendon be zero:

$$\text{Force}_{\text{Muscle}} + \text{Force}_{\text{Tendon}} = 0$$
$$50 \text{ N} + \text{Force}_{\text{Tendon}} = 0$$
$$\text{Force}_{\text{Tendon}} = -50 \text{ N}$$

So the force on the transverse section of the tendon must also have a magnitude of 50 newtons, but in the opposite direction as the muscle force.

We can measure the cross-section of the tendon and find it to be approximately rectangular in shape, with dimensions of 1 by 4 millimeters. The stress on the transverse section of the tendon is the force divided by the cross-sectional area:

$$\text{Stress} = \frac{50 \text{ N}}{0.001 \text{ m} \times 0.004 \text{ m}}$$
$$= 12.5 \text{ MPa}$$

Since the tendon is of uniform cross-section throughout most of its length, the examination of the next segment of tendon will reveal a 12.5-megapascal stress at the most distal cross-sectional area as well.

What would be the stress on the internal longitudinal surface of the tendon (Fig. 4.4)? We will apply the equilibrium principle that states that the sum of the forces must equal zero. The intensity of the load (the stress) is 12.5 megapascals. Since we now have created a transverse surface measuring 1 by

2 millimeters, half the area of the original tendon, the force on the proximal transverse cross-section must be:

$$\text{Force} = \text{Stress} \times \text{Area}$$
$$= 12.5 \text{ MPa} \times (0.001 \text{ m} \times 0.002 \text{ m})$$
$$= 25 \text{ N}$$

This force must be the same as the force at the distal end of the tendon because of equilibrium. As there are no other forces applied to the free outer longitudinal surface of the tendon, and the sum of the two forces applied at the two transverse surfaces equals zero, there can be no force applied to the imagined midsurface longitudinal plane. Thus, we see that the stress on the tendon's internal longitudinal surface must be zero.

As we will see later in this chapter, tendon as a material is capable of sustaining a stress of 12.5 megapascals without damage. This, of course, is true only for the stresses applied on the *transverse surfaces* of the tendon. As anyone familiar with the structure of a tendon is aware, the longitudinal surfaces of a tendon can sustain virtually no stress; any attempt to impose such a stress results in fiber separation. Thus, the application of equilibrium principles, coupled with the definition of stress, produces results consistent with our intuitive knowledge of tendon material.

## Shear Stress

As we previously described, shear stress is the condition that exists when the force applied to a material's surface is oriented parallel to that surface. When long bones are subjected to twisting loads about their long axis, shear stresses develop in the bone tissue. This common loading situation, termed torsional loading, will be examined in more detail in Chapter 5. However, we will use an example here of the tibia under conditions of torsional load (Fig. 4.5).

If we externally rotate the foot, a twisting moment (torque) will induce forces on the proximal surface of the tibial segment that produce the moment necessary to maintain equilibrium in the distal segment. This moment (torque) will tend to internally rotate the tibial segment. The forces that produce this moment act parallel to the transverse surface of the tibia in a counterclockwise direction. If we examine a small piece of bone (Fig. 4.5), we see that the upper surface of the piece is subjected to a portion of the force creating the internal resisting torque. This force, acting on the upper transverse surface, produces a shear stress.

Let's consider the small piece of bone as an object in equilibrium. If we had only the one force acting on the upper surface of the object, the sum of the forces in the horizontal direction would not be zero. To balance the force on the upper surface, we can visualize a force on the lower surface of the piece of equal intensity, but opposite in direction. The sum of the two forces on the upper and lower surfaces will satisfy equilibrium (Equation 1.3) in the horizontal direction.

If we consider rotational equilibrium (Equation 1.4) by summing the moments about the center of the piece of bone, we see that each of the two forces

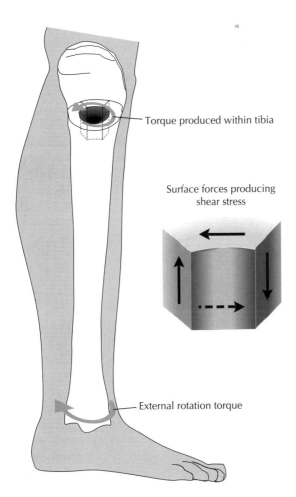

Torque produced within tibia

Surface forces producing
shear stress

External rotation torque

**Figure 4.5.** External rotation of the foot is resisted within the tibia by a torque generated by forces acting parallel to the transverse plane of the tibia. These forces produce shear stress on the transverse cross-section.

produces a clockwise moment. Thus, the sum of the moments cannot be zero. The piece cannot be held in equilibrium without some additional imposed forces. These additional forces are applied to the longitudinal surfaces, again in directions parallel to these surfaces. The directions of these forces, upward on the right surface and downward on the left surface, provide a counterclockwise moment. Since the intensity of these forces is the same as the intensity of the horizontal forces, moment equilibrium is achieved. Note also that because the two forces on the longitudinal surfaces are equal in magnitude, force equilibrium in the longitudinal direction is also maintained.

From our definition of shear stress, the condition on the transverse and longitudinal faces of the cube of bone from the tibia is a shear stress. Thus, we see that applying torsional loads to long bones produces shear stress on both transverse surfaces and longitudinal surfaces within the bone. These shear stresses are of equal intensity. The condition of equal-intensity shear stresses on four faces of a cube of material is known as pure shear. It is the simplest shear stress configuration, just as our example of the tendon being stretched is the simplest tension stress configuration. Note that whereas there were no stresses on the tendon's longitudinal surfaces under the application of simple tensile stress, there are shear stresses on the bone's longitudinal surfaces under the application of pure shear stress.

Shear stresses usually exist in all structures that are carrying loads. The bone plate in Figure 4.6 has been fastened to a set of grips and has 500 newtons of load applied in the longitudinal direction. Consider the bottom segment of the plate and grip, and realize that it must be in equilibrium. The segment's top transverse surface must be carrying a 500-newton load if equilibrium is to be satisfied in the longitudinal direction (Equation 1.3). The normal stress produced by this 500-newton force may be calculated from Equation 4.2:

$$\text{Normal stress} = \frac{F_\perp}{\text{Area}}$$

$$= \frac{500 \text{ N}}{4.17 \text{ mm} \times 12 \text{ mm}}$$

$$= 10 \text{ MPa}$$

We will now consider a segment of the plate, formed by passing an imaginary oblique plane through the plate's center (Fig. 4.6). We previously calculated the force on the lower transverse surface to be 500 newtons. In order for the plate segment to be in equilibrium, the upper oblique surface must also have sufficient stress intensity to produce a 500-newton longitudinal force. If we now resolve the 500-newton force into two components, one parallel to the oblique surface and one perpendicular to the surface, we see that according to our definitions, the oblique surface will have both normal stress and shear stress.

Let's calculate the intensity of these stresses. If the oblique surface is oriented at 45 degrees to the transverse surface, then the oblique surface area is related to the transverse surface area:

$$\text{Area}_{\text{Oblique}} = \frac{\text{Area}_{\text{Trans}}}{\sin 45°}$$

$$= \frac{50 \text{ mm}^2}{0.707}$$

$$= 70.7 \text{ mm}^2$$

Similarly, the force component perpendicular to the transverse surface is

$$\text{Force}_\perp = \text{Force} \times \sin 45°$$

$$= 500 \text{ N} \times 0.707$$

$$= 353.5 \text{ N}$$

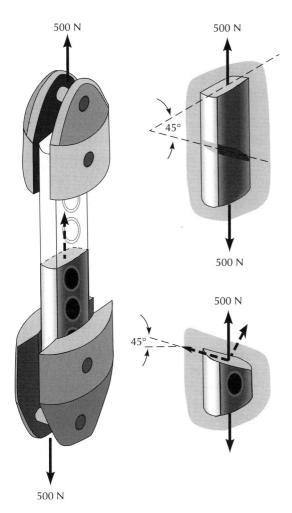

**Figure 4.6.** A 316L stainless steel bone plate is gripped and loaded in tension by a 500-newton load. A free body is formed from the lower grip and lower portion of the plate. A second free body is formed by passing a boundary through the center of the plate at an angle of 45 degrees to the plate's long axis and then transversely through the bottom of the plate.

Thus, the normal stress on the oblique surface is (from Equation 4.2):

$$\text{Normal stress}_{\text{Oblique}} = \frac{353.5 \text{ N}}{70.7 \text{ mm}^2}$$

$$= 5 \text{ MPa}$$

Note that this value is one-half the normal stress on the transverse surface.

The force component parallel to the oblique surface has the same magnitude as the perpendicular component:

$$\text{Force}_{\parallel} = \text{Force} \times \cos 45°$$

$$= 500 \text{ N} \times 0.707$$

$$= 353.5 \text{ N}$$

Thus, the shear stress on the oblique surface is also 5 megapascals, half the intensity of the normal stress on the transverse surface.

In fact, whenever an object with a uniform cross-section is under tensile loading, planes oriented obliquely to the load carry both shear and tensile stresses. The plane with the largest tensile stress is the transverse plane. This plane has no shear stress. The planes with the largest shear stress are oblique planes oriented at 45 degrees to the loading axis. The magnitude of the highest shear stress is one-half the magnitude of the highest tensile stress.

## STRAIN

In the simple example that we have presented, we were able to calculate stress with relative ease. In most situations involving biological structures, the object's shape and composition do not lend themselves to such a simple, direct calculation of stress. The structure may be composed of several materials and be of such a complex geometry as to make it difficult to use the principles of equilibrium to determine internal forces. This was certainly the case, for example, in Chapter 1, when we considered the problem of calculating forces about a joint when more than one muscle contraction occurred across the joint.

In such cases, we need a measurement tool that provides for direct observations of physical phenomena that can be correlated to the existence of stresses. It has long been recognized that when loads are applied to an object, the object deforms in response to the loads. Thus, a methodology has been developed whereby the deformations are correlated with the stress intensities produced by the applied loads.

### Normal Strain

Let's examine how a simple structure deforms under load. Consider the stainless steel bone plate that we first examined in the discussion of combined shear and normal stresses. The bone plate in Figure 4.7 has again been fastened to a set of grips and is being loaded in the longitudinal direction. In addition to measuring the load, we have applied an instrument called an extensometer to the midsection of the plate. The extensometer measures the change in distance between its two attachment points on the plate. As we apply load, we

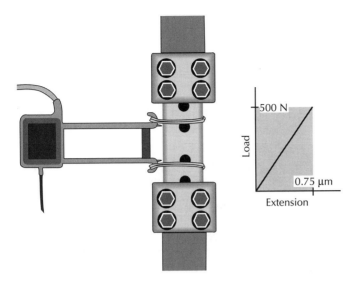

**Figure 4.7.** An extensometer, used to measure the change in distance between the two attachment points, has been fastened to the central portion of the bone plate from Figure 4.6. The accompanying graph shows the load applied to the plate plotted against the resulting extension experienced by the plate (as measured by the extensometer).

will record and plot both the load (on the vertical axis of a graph) and the extension sensed by the extensometer (on the horizontal axis). As we apply the load, we notice that the curve produced on the graph is a straight line. When the load reaches 500 newtons, we measure an extension between the points of the extensometer of 0.00075 millimeters, or 0.75 micrometers ($\mu$m). The prefix *micro* ($\mu$) means one-millionth. At this point, we release the load, and the curve is retraced back to the origin. Repeating the loading process up to 500 newtons reproduces the original curve.

This experiment allows us to make some general observations and to formulate some definitions. Based on our previous example (Fig. 4.6), the stress on the transverse surface is 10 megapascals. Corresponding to the 500-newton load, we observed 0.75 micrometers of elongation in the plate's central portion. This elongation took place between measuring points of the extensometer that were spaced 15 millimeters (15,000 micrometers) apart (Fig. 4.7). Therefore, each micrometer of plate length experienced an elongation of $5 \times 10^{-5}$ micrometers. We define this *ratio of elongation to unit length as tensile strain.* Had we done a compressive test on the plate, in which the loads are applied in the opposite direction, a shortening of the unit length of the plate would have occurred. We define *the ratio of shortening to unit length as compressive strain.*

Tensile and compressive strains are grouped into a single classification termed *normal strain.* Thus, the definition of *normal strain* is

$$\text{Normal strain} = \frac{\text{Change in length}}{\text{Unit length}} \qquad (4.3)$$

It may be a positive quantity (tensile strain) or a negative quantity (compressive strain). In both the tensile and compressive cases, strain has no units, since it is the ratio of two quantities both in units of length. In our example, the 316L-type stainless steel bone plate displays a tensile strain (from Equation 4.3) of

$$\text{Tensile strain} = \frac{0.75 \ \mu\text{m}}{15,000 \ \mu\text{m}}$$

$$= 50 \times 10^{-6}$$

when subjected to a 10-megapascal stress. Because strains are often very small quantities, it is common to express strain using the unit of microstrain. In our example, the 0.75-micrometer elongation created a tensile strain of 50 microstrain.

### Shear Strain

Returning to our example of the tibia under torsional loading, we observe that when the foot is externally rotated under a torsional load of 10 newton-meters, the distal tibia externally rotates with respect to the proximal tibia. Simple measurement of the proximal tibia relative to the distal tibia reveals a rotational displacement of 3 degrees. The small piece of bone tissue (Fig. 4.8) within the tibia undergoes a similar distortion, but on a smaller scale. The longitudinal edges are now oriented in a slightly oblique direction, so that there are no longer any right (90-degree) angles between the sides of the piece. *This change in angle between the two faces of the piece of bone that were formerly oriented at 90 degrees to one another is defined as shear strain.* In this case, the change in each angle between the faces is 0.05 degrees. While we often measure changes in angle in units of degrees, by convention shear strain is always expressed in units of radians (discussed in Chapter 1). The change in angle of 0.05 degrees corresponds to a shear strain of 0.000915 radians ($915 \times 10^{-6}$ radians).

**Figure 4.8.** The torque applied to the tibia (Fig. 4.5) causes shear strain in the small piece of bone tissue.

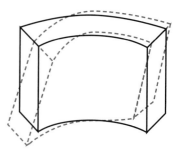

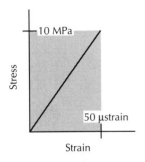

**Figure 4.9.** The plot of stress versus strain for the 316L stainless steel material of the bone plate is a straight line with a slope of 200 gigapascals.

## MODULUS OF ELASTICITY

As we noted previously, loading and unloading the bone plate demonstrates a constant linear relationship between load and extension (Fig. 4.7). We will use this tensile test to illustrate some important definitions of material properties. Because the load-versus-elongation curve is fully reversible, we say that the material behaves elastically. *Elastic behavior implies that when the load is released, there is no permanent change in the shape of the structure.* All of the shape changes induced by the applied load disappear when the load is released.

It is possible to take every point on the load-versus-extension curve (Fig. 4.7) and calculate the corresponding stress (Equation 4.1) and strain (Equation 4.3). We may then plot these points as a stress-versus-strain curve (Fig. 4.9). We observe that the relationship between the calculated stress and the measured strain is linear (the slope of the line is constant). For our example of the stainless steel bone plate, the value of the ratio is

$$\frac{\text{Stress}}{\text{Strain}} = \frac{10 \text{ MPa}}{50 \text{ microstrain}}$$

$$= \frac{10 \times 10^6 \text{ Pa}}{50 \times 10^{-6}}$$

$$= 200 \times 10^9 \text{ Pa}$$

$$= 200 \text{ GPa}$$

where the unit gigapascal (GPa) is equal to one billion ($10^9$) pascals. If we conduct many such tension or compression experiments on different sizes and shapes of stainless steel specimens, we will find that this ratio does not change. Regardless of the size and shape, the ratio of tensile stress to tensile strain remains the same.

The ratio of stress to strain depends, therefore, on the material being tested and not on the shape of the structure being tested. *This ratio is termed the modulus of elasticity,* and it is also often called the elastic modulus or Young's modulus, after the English scientist, Thomas Young. It is usually denoted by the letter $E$:

$$\text{Modulus of elasticity} = E = \frac{\text{Normal stress}}{\text{Normal strain}} \qquad (4.4)$$

The modulus of elasticity is constant for each material and is thus a measure of the material's ability to maintain shape under the application of external loads. Materials with high elastic moduli are stiffer and more resistant to deformation for any particular shape and loading than materials with lower elastic moduli.

Consider again our example of the tendon (Fig. 4.3). Let's repeat the observation of the tendon when it is loaded by the pull of the muscle contraction. This time we will mark the tendon with two transverse lines spaced 10 millimeters apart, and we will observe the separation of the lines while the muscle applies load to the tendon. As in our bone plate example, we will plot a graph of load versus the separation distance of the two lines.

When the load reaches 50 newtons, the lines are observed to have separated a distance of 0.2 millimeters (200 micrometers). Remembering that the cross-sectional area of the tendon was 4 square millimeters, we can now calculate the modulus of elasticity for tendon material (from Equation 4.4):

$$E_{\text{Tendon}} = \frac{\left(\dfrac{50\ \text{N}}{4\ \text{mm}^2}\right)}{\left(\dfrac{0.2\ \text{mm}}{10\ \text{mm}}\right)}$$

$$= \frac{12.5\ \text{MPa}}{20{,}000\ \text{microstrain}}$$

$$= 625\ \text{MPa}$$

Note that this modulus of elasticity is much lower than that observed for 316L-type stainless steel. We note, therefore, that tendon as a material is much less stiff than stainless steel. Both materials exhibit elastic behavior, in that removal of the load results in restoration of the original length of the tendon structure and of the bone plate.

## MODULUS OF RIGIDITY

If we return to the example of the tibia that is being externally rotated, observation will reveal that upon release of the torsional load, the tibia returns to its initial configuration. Thus, when the induced shear stresses in the material return to zero, the distortions (the shear strains) also return to zero. We have defined such behavior as elastic. If we plot a graph of shear stress versus shear strain during loading and unloading of the tibia, we would see linear, reversible behavior. Thus, for each change in shear stress, there is a corresponding proportional change in shear strain. *The ratio of shear stress to shear strain is termed the modulus of rigidity or the shear modulus* and is usually denoted by the letter $G$:

$$\text{Shear modulus} = G = \frac{\text{Shear stress}}{\text{Shear strain}} \qquad (4.5)$$

Like the modulus of elasticity, the modulus of rigidity is a property of the material that may be thought of as a measure of the resistance of the material to distortion when placed under load. A typical loading situation that produces distortion is torsional loading; therefore, the shear modulus is a comparative measure of the ability of the material to provide resistance against distortion under torsional load.

Consider the segment of tibial bone (Fig. 4.8). The shear stress was calculated earlier to be 3 megapascals, corresponding to a shear strain of 0.000915 radians. This corresponds to a shear modulus for bone tissue of

$$G_{\text{Bone}} = \frac{3 \text{ MPa}}{0.000915 \text{ radians}}$$

$$= 3.3 \text{ GPa}$$

If we made an exact model of the tibia from poly(methyl methacrylate) (PMMA), a material with a shear modulus of 1.1 gigapascals, the angulation induced by the same 10-newton-meter torque would be three times (3.3 GPa/1.1 GPa) that induced in the natural tibia.

## POISSON'S EFFECT

Simple material tensile tests reveal that associated with the tensile strain in the loading direction is a compressive strain perpendicular to the loading direction. Stretching a rubber band, for example, and observing the simultaneous reduction in width and thickness of the band as it stretches will verify this phenomenon. The same result occurs in stretching biological materials, such as tendon, ligament, and muscle. It is, in fact, a universal phenomenon observed in all materials—metals, bone tissue, plastics, ceramics, and even liquids. This phenomenon is termed *Poisson's effect*, after the French mathematician, Siméon Poisson.

Poisson's effect is the third type of elastic behavior exhibited by materials. The effect is quantified by observing the strain magnitude in the direction perpendicular to loading and comparing this to the strain magnitude in the direction of loading. Consider again the example of the stainless steel bone plate used in our discussion of normal strain. If we placed an extensometer in the transverse direction to measure the change in width of the plate, upon application of the 500-newton tensile load, the 12-millimeter-wide plate would decrease in width by 0.18 micrometers. This means that the normal strain in the transverse direction is (from Equation 4.3)

$$\text{Strain}_{\text{Trans}} = \frac{-0.18 \ \mu m}{12 \times 10^{-3} \ m}$$

$$= -15 \text{ microstrain}$$

Remembering that the longitudinal strain in the bone plate caused by the 500-newton load was 50 microstrain, *the ratio of transverse to longitudinal strain* for stainless steel can be calculated. This ratio is called *Poisson's ratio* and is denoted by the Greek letter $\nu$:

$$\text{Poisson's ratio} = \nu = \frac{\text{Strain}_{\text{Trans}}}{\text{Strain}_{\text{Long}}}$$

$$= \frac{-15 \text{ microstrain}}{50 \text{ microstrain}}$$

$$= 0.3$$

The negative sign is usually omitted in reporting Poisson's ratio. This is a commonly accepted value for this property for most metallic materials, and the value is only slightly different for other types of materials. In general, Poisson's ratio is less than 0.5. This simply means that a material's volume under simple tensile load cannot diminish, and that a material's volume under simple compressive load cannot increase.

Just as in our example of the tendon, where we found no stresses on the longitudinal surfaces, there is no stress on the longitudinal surfaces of the plate. Though planes in other orientations with respect to the loading axis contained stresses, there were no stresses corresponding to the transverse compressive strain observed across the width of the plate. Thus, compressive strain in a transverse direction does not correlate with a compressive stress. The transverse compressive strain is, in fact, a response of the material to longitudinal tensile strain rather than a response to an induced stress.

## RELATION BETWEEN THE ELASTIC PROPERTIES

We have now defined three elastic properties for a material: the modulus of elasticity, the modulus of rigidity, and Poisson's ratio. To examine the relation between these properties, let's repeat our example of stretching the tendon under a 50-newton load. This time, we will draw a square on the surface of the tendon so that the diagonals of the square lie along the longitudinal and transverse directions (Fig. 4.10). When we apply the load, the longitudinal diagonal undergoes 20,000 microstrain. The transverse diagonal, because of Poisson's effect, undergoes 6000 microstrain (assuming Poisson's ratio for tendon to be 0.3).

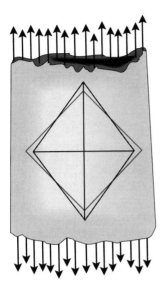

**Figure 4.10.** A diamond drawn on the tendon from Figure 4.3 shows distortion and elongation under the influence of the applied tensile load.

Just as there is a relation between the amount of normal tensile stress and the shear stress that exists on transverse and diagonal planes (as we discussed earlier in this chapter), so there is a relation between normal strain and shear strain. The angle of the distorted square on the tendon under the 50-newton load can be calculated from the lengths of the two diagonals. The change in length of the longitudinal diagonal depends only on the elastic modulus:

$$\text{Change in length} \propto \frac{1}{E}$$

The change in length of the transverse diagonal depends only on Poisson's ratio:

$$\text{Change in length} \propto \nu$$

Thus, the change in angle (that is, the shear strain) can be expressed in terms of these two elastic constants ($E$ and $\nu$).

The shear modulus was defined as the ratio of shear stress to shear strain (Equation 4.5), and, as we showed previously for a simple tension test, the shear stress is related to tensile stress. Therefore, the shear modulus must be related to the tensile stress and the other two elastic constants. But the tensile stress is related to the normal strain (occurring along the longitudinal diagonal) and the elastic modulus. Substituting into Equation 4.5 for the shear stress in terms of the tensile stress and for the shear strain in terms of the other two elastic constants, the shear modulus becomes

$$\text{Shear modulus} = \frac{E}{2 \times (1 + \nu)}$$

Thus, every material has three elastic properties, but only two of these properties are independent of the third. If the elastic modulus and Poisson's ratio are obtained from a tension test, a simple calculation will reveal the shear modulus for the material. Thus, a simple tension test of bone tissue can be used to quantify bone's resistance to angular distortion under torsional loading.

## STRAIN ENERGY

In Chapter 2 we introduced the concept of *work as a force moving through a distance* and the concept of *energy as a potential for doing work.* Let's apply these two concepts to our example of loading a stainless steel bone plate. We wish to find the work required to elongate the central 15-millimeter segment of the plate when the 500-newton load is applied. Imagine, in our example, that the upper transverse surface of the plate at the level of the extensometer is held fixed. When we apply the 500-newton tensile force to the bottom of the plate, the lower transverse plate surface at the bottom level of the extensometer moves 0.75 micrometers, as we saw before. The plot of force versus extension demonstrates that as the force is applied, the point of application of the force (the lower transverse surface) moves. To calculate the amount of work done by the tensile force, we can multiply each force increment by each extension increment. This process will give us the area under the force-extension curve.

Thus, for the plate material between the extensometer attachment points, the tensile force does an amount of work equal to the area of the triangle formed by the force-versus-extension plot:

$$\text{Area of triangle} = \tfrac{1}{2} \times \text{Height} \times \text{Base}$$

$$\text{Work} = \tfrac{1}{2} \times \text{Force} \times \text{Extension}$$

$$= \tfrac{1}{2} \times 500 \text{ N} \times 0.75 \text{ } \mu\text{m}$$

$$= 0.000188 \text{ N} \cdot \text{m}$$

$$= 0.000188 \text{ J}$$

Because the loading cycle is reversible, this stored energy is available to do work during the unloading cycle. The lower plate surface has the capability of raising a force varying from 500 newtons to 0 newtons through an extension height of 0.75 micrometers. The energy stored in the plate is called strain energy. *All objects that are loaded will deform, and the resulting energy put into the object is strain energy.* If the object is composed of an elastic material, the strain energy is further defined as *elastic strain energy.* Elastic strain energy is recoverable when the object returns to its original shape.

One biological tissue is particularly efficient at storing elastic strain energy. This material is known as elastin, and its force-versus-extension curve is definitively linear and reversible. One creature takes advantage of elastin in its unique form of locomotion. The flea uses a band of elastin fibers that crosses the joints of the rear limbs as a means of propulsion. Before jumping, the flea rotates the joint so that the elastin fibers are fully stretched, and the joint is held in an overextended, stable position. This extension of the elastin fibers by relatively slow muscle action allows the elastin material to store strain energy. A small muscle force is then exerted to unlock the joint by moving it over center when the flea decides to jump. The elastic strain energy stored in the elastin fibers is rapidly dissipated and transformed into kinetic energy, a process that is much quicker than muscle contraction. The result is that the flea can jump much faster and farther than would be possible by active muscle contraction.

## STATIC LOAD BEHAVIOR

The concepts of stress and strain enable us to describe the burden imposed upon materials that comprise both natural and artificial structures. To predict the limits of performance of these structures, we must investigate the limits of performance of the materials from which they are made. To do this, we will apply the concepts just developed to explain and categorize the empirically observed performance of materials under extreme loading conditions.

Let's begin by performing a simple tension test on a piece of cortical bone tissue. We remove the piece of tissue from the cortex of the femoral diaphysis and cut it into an appropriate shape (Fig. 4.11), so that the long axis of the specimen is parallel to the longitudinal axis of the femur. We place the specimen in a machine capable of exerting tensile force and simultaneously record the magnitude of the force and the elongation of the central portion of the specimen (as measured by the extensometer). From the measured force and

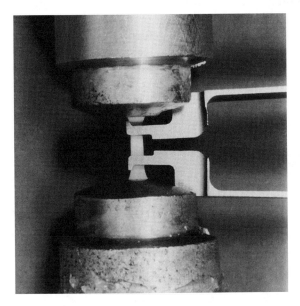

**Figure 4.11.** A standardized bone specimen cut from the diaphysis of a femur is loaded in tension with an extensometer attached to measure change in length.

the area of the specimen, we can calculate the stress, and from the measured change in length and the original length between the knife edges of the extensometer, we can calculate the strain. As we continue to apply increasing tensile force until the specimen ruptures, we produce a stress-versus-strain curve (Fig. 4.12). Notice that this curve has two distinct regions composed of nearly straight lines with a curved transition region joining them.

Let's take a second specimen and load it up to point *A* on the curve (near the end of the first linear region) and then remove the load. The bone tissue exhibits reversible or elastic behavior and returns to its original, unloaded length. The loading curve, although not perfectly straight, is usually approximated as a straight line. As we've already discussed in this chapter, the slope of the line is called the elastic modulus. A typical value for elastic modulus is 18 gigapascals.

The test results described for our cortical bone specimen are based upon loading the specimen in a direction corresponding to the long axis of the femur from which the specimen was cut. If the bone tissue specimen is oriented in another direction (for example, parallel to the transverse direction in the bone), the test results will be quite different (Fig. 4.12). The curve has one linear region and a short transition to the rupture point. While the initial elastic region is qualitatively similar to that observed on the longitudinal specimen, the slope of this region (that is, the elastic modulus) is only about two-thirds as great as for the longitudinal direction. Thus, the modulus of elasticity of bone tissue strongly depends on specimen orientation. *Materials whose properties vary with loading direction are called anisotropic materials.*

Bone tissue specimens have also been tested under torsional load to determine the modulus of rigidity (*G*). Small cylindrical specimens are placed in a machine that applies a torsional load and simultaneously measures the applied load and the angular deformation that the specimen undergoes. The initial straight-line portion of the resulting torque-versus-deformation curve is used to calculate *G*. A typical value for bone tissue is 6.9 gigapascals.

Artificial materials are often used to reinforce or replace diseased or damaged bone tissue. Analyses to determine the loads that structures made from such a material can withstand require knowledge of the material's elastic modulus. Let's examine the contrasting behavior of two "plastics" commonly used

**Figure 4.12.** Plots of tension stress versus strain for cortical bone tissue tested along both the long axis of the bone and the transverse axis of the bone (1).

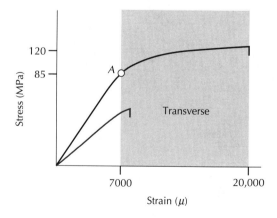

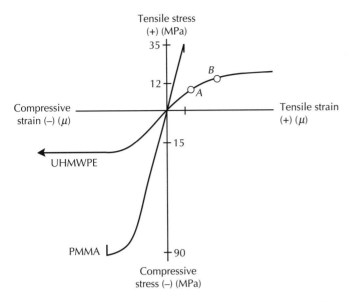

**Figure 4.13.** Stress-versus-strain curves in both tension and compression for PMMA and UHMWPE. The elastic modulus of PMMA is about 3 gigapascals, and the modulus of UHMWPE is about 1 gigapascal (2, 3).

in total-joint replacement. PMMA is used as a load-bearing grout material to fix implants to the surrounding bone. If we mold a test specimen from PMMA and then load it in tension and compression, we produce a stress-versus-strain curve (Fig. 4.13). While the tensile and compressive portions of the curve are not identical, the slopes of both portions (the elastic moduli) are the same.

The other commonly used "plastic" is ultra-high-molecular-weight polyethylene (UHMWPE). It is used as a bearing material in virtually all total joint replacements. Tensile and compression tests of polyethylene specimens produce highly nonlinear stress-versus-strain curves (Fig. 4.13). Examination reveals an approximately linear initial portion to both curves. Unlike PMMA, different UHMWPE formulations have different elastic moduli. Of particular importance is the extreme dependence of the modulus on the density of the material. For example, a change in density from 0.935 to 0.955 grams/centimeter$^3$ corresponds to a change in modulus from 1.0 to 1.6 gigapascals. Such density variations occur from radiation sterilization and subsequent aging.

If our analysis for a particular problem is concerned with loading polyethylene in such a way as to produce relatively low stresses, as occur in the initial portion of the curve, then we can designate the slope of this portion as the elastic modulus. However, the *in vivo* loads experienced by total-joint-replacement components often produce stresses beyond those in the initial, straight-line portion of the curve. What value of elastic modulus is appropriate, for example, in an analysis in which the stresses correspond to those between points *A* and *B* in Figure 4.13?

There are two common methods for assigning an elastic modulus to a region of nonlinear stress-versus-strain behavior in a material. The first method is the

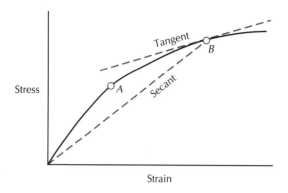

**Figure 4.14.** Elastic modulus for a material with nonlinear stress-versus-strain behavior is commonly assigned in one of two ways, using either the secant or the tangent method.

**Table 4.1.** Elastic Moduli of Common Orthopaedic Materials (4)

| Material | $E$ (GPa) |
| --- | --- |
| $Al_2O_3$ | 550 |
| Cobalt alloy | 200 |
| Stainless steel | 180 |
| Titanium alloy | 110 |
| Bone tissue | 18 |
| PMMA | 3 |
| UHMWPE | 1 |

secant method, in which the elastic modulus is taken as the slope of a line from the origin to the point in question (Fig. 4.14). This method underestimates the elastic modulus at low stresses and overestimates the modulus at high stresses. It is useful in analyses that attempt to predict the performance of the material in devices that have large load variations. A typical example of an analysis in which the secant method would be used is calculating the deflection of a polyethylene tibial component from a total knee replacement under regular loading conditions.

The second method for determining elastic modulus in a material behaving nonlinearly is the tangent method, in which the modulus is taken as the slope of a line drawn tangent to the stress-versus-strain curve at the point of interest (Fig. 4.14). This approximation is useful in analyses concerned with the effects of small load variations about some relatively high mean load value. An example of an analysis in which the tangent method would be used is determining the stress variation induced in the articulating surface of a polyethylene tibial plateau component during the stance phase of normal gait.

We can now compare the elastic moduli from the materials that we have examined in this chapter (Table 4.1). Note that there are large differences due to the very different molecular structures of these materials. Stainless steel, for example, has an ordered, crystalline structure, with the atoms held together by strong metallic bonds. In contrast, polyethylene is made up of long polymer chains, with the atoms along the chain held together by strong covalent bonds, but with the chains themselves attracted to each other by much weaker hydrogen bonds. The elastic modulus is critically dependent on the type of atomic or molecular bonding and the structure of the material at the atomic level.

## HYSTERESIS

If we load a cortical bone specimen in a cyclic manner with progressively higher loads, we will create a highly nonlinear stress-versus-strain curve (Fig. 4.15). When we load the bone specimen up to point $A$ and then remove the load, the specimen exhibits reversible behavior and returns to its original, unloaded length. Note that the loading and unloading curves do not overlap. Rather, they form a closed loop, known as a *hysteresis loop*. Such behavior is typical of biological materials. A hysteresis loop can be thought of as an inefficiency in the process of storing and releasing strain energy. As we discussed previously in this chapter, the area under the loading curve represents the strain energy stored in the material during loading. The area under the unloading curve represents the release of strain energy during unloading. The difference in area under the two curves, the area enclosed within the hysteresis loop, represents the energy dissipated within the material. This energy is dissipated primarily by two processes: mechanical damage to the material and internal friction. For bone tissue, each loading cycle induces both processes. The effect of mechanical damage to bone tissue will be more fully considered in Chapter 6.

Like bone tissue, most "plastics" exhibit hysteresis. These materials are typically composed of very long, intertwined polymer chains. Within such a structure under load, there is ample opportunity for internal friction between chains. This can be contrasted with metallic materials, which typically have a very crystalline, ordered structure with fewer mechanisms for generating internal friction or for experiencing damage at low stresses. Metallic materials, therefore, do not typically exhibit a hysteresis loop as part of their stress-versus-strain behavior.

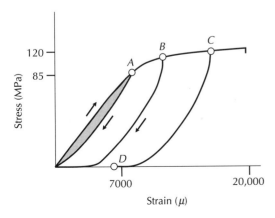

**Figure 4.15.** When the specimen is loaded to point $A$ and the load is released, the bone immediately returns to its original length, although not along the same path as the loading process. When the specimen is loaded to point $B$ and released, the elongation does not immediately return to zero. It requires several seconds at zero load for the specimen to return to its original length. Loading to point $C$ produces a change in length that is not reversible.

**Figure 4.16.** Three stress-versus-strain curves for cortical bone tissue tested in tension at three different rates. As the testing rate increases, note that the slope (the elastic modulus) of the initial, straight-line portion increases.

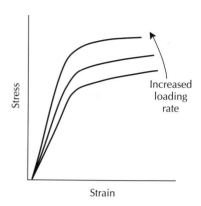

## VISCOELASTICITY

Now let's load the cortical bone tissue specimen beyond point *A* to point *B* in Figure 4.15 and again release the load. We observe that the loading and unloading curves do not immediately form a closed loop. However, if we allow some time to pass after unloading the bone specimen, the bone tissue will regain its original length. *When the behavior of a material depends upon the time conditions associated with loading and unloading, the material is said to be viscoelastic.*

To further illustrate this phenomenon, let's test a series of three additional longitudinal cortical bone tissue specimens, but let's apply the tensile force to each specimen at a different rate. Figure 4.16 shows the curves for the three specimens, with loading to rupture accomplished in 1 second, 0.1 second, and 0.01 second. The elastic moduli are noticeably different for the three specimens, increasing with the loading rate. This is typical for viscoelastic materials, though the sensitivity of the modulus to loading rate will vary. For example, mechanical testing of ligaments has revealed that, unlike bone tissue, ligament material exhibits little viscoelastic behavior. Thus, the elastic modulus of ligament material does not depend significantly on how fast load is applied to the ligament.

We can again contrast the "plastics" and metallic materials with respect to viscoelastic behavior. Plastic materials are typically viscoelastic, with mechanical properties that vary with the loading rate. Metallic materials, on the other hand, do not typically exhibit viscoelastic behavior. The mechanical properties of metallic materials do not change appreciably with the loading rate. The difference in viscoelastic behavior between "plastics" and metals can be explained by their molecular structure in the same manner as was used to describe differences in the hysteresis between these two types of materials.

## FAILURE CRITERIA

While some biomechanical analyses seek to determine the deformations imposed by loads (for example, motion of the bone fragments at a fracture site treated by an external fixator), others seek knowledge of the maximum load that can be safely carried (for example, the load required to permanently deform a hip nail-plate device). The first set of problems requires knowledge of the elastic properties of the materials involved in the structures being considered, and the second set of problems requires knowledge of the failure criteria of the materials.

How do we characterize the material properties that define failure? Let's reexamine the stress-versus-strain curve measured from the cortical bone tissue specimen (Fig. 4.15) and consider the second region of the curve. Unlike loading and unloading in the initial elastic or reversible region, loading and unloading in the second region results in permanent changes in the material. If, for example, we load the specimen up to point $C$ and then remove the load, the bone tissue never returns to its original size; there is a residual or permanent deformation (denoted as point $D$). We customarily describe this region of the stress-versus-strain curve as the *inelastic* (sometimes called *plastic*) region.

To experience sufficient stress to reach the inelastic region, the bone tissue must undergo permanent structural change caused by some form of mechanical damage. This is easily seen for bone tissue that is loaded in compression. In this mode of loading, bone tissue is able to sustain a stress of about 190 megapascals before entering the inelastic region of the stress-versus-strain curve. Continued loading beyond this stress produces macroscopically visible, oblique disruption patterns that, when examined microscopically, show a complex failure geometry (Fig. 4.17). While structural changes also occur in the inelastic region under tensile loading conditions, these changes are not as apparent because they are at an ultrastructural (crystalline) level.

For bone tissue and other materials that first exhibit elastic and then exhibit inelastic behavior, there are two separate conditions for which failure

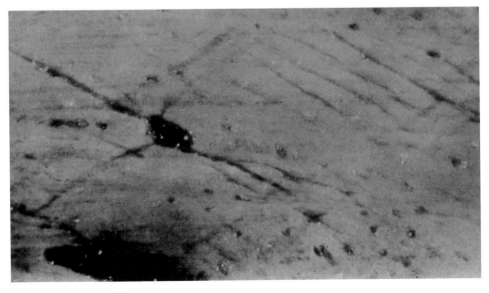

**Figure 4.17.** Cortical bone tissue overloaded in compression exhibits mechanical damage in the form of cracks.

criteria may be appropriately obtained. The first is the transition between elastic (reversible) behavior and inelastic behavior (where permanent damage is initiated). The second condition is the point of rupture of the material. Some problem solutions require knowledge of damage initiation. Two typical examples are the determination of the maximum tolerable load that can be imposed upon the tibia before initiation of "stress fractures," and the determination of the maximum load that can be imposed upon a hip nail-plate before it permanently deforms. Solutions to other problems, such as the torque required to produce a spiral fracture of the tibia or the joint reaction force needed to fracture a PMMA cement mantle around a femoral component of a total hip replacement, require knowledge of the material's rupture strength. These two failure criteria are usually expressed in terms of the stress corresponding to the transition point. In the first criterion, *the stress at the transition point of the stress-versus-strain curve between the elastic and inelastic regions is termed the yield stress.* In the second criterion, *the stress at the point of rupture of the material is called the ultimate stress.* Typical values of these criteria for the materials we've been considering are given in Table 4.2.

Not all materials exhibit separate yield and ultimate stresses. For example, when PMMA is loaded in tension (Fig. 4.13), failure occurs within the elastic region. Thus, PMMA exhibits no inelastic region and, therefore, no yield stress. The stress at failure is the ultimate stress. *Materials that do not exhibit an inelastic region are called brittle materials.* Rupture of a brittle material produces a fracture pattern that allows reassembly of the fragments into the original shape. You can restore broken pottery, for example, to the original shape, with sufficient patience, by gluing the pieces back together. Thus, ceramics used for pottery are brittle materials. Restoring a crushed tin can to its original shape is not nearly as easy, because large, permanent shape changes have occurred in the metal.

The two failure criteria (stress criteria) that we have identified are not the only criteria that can be chosen. Consider, for example, a stress-versus-strain curve produced from tensile loading of three common implant metals: stainless steel, cobalt alloy, and titanium alloy. Each of these metallic materials exhibits a different stress-versus-strain curve, and each has a yield stress and ultimate

**Table 4.2.** Yield and Ultimate Stresses for Common Orthopaedic Materials (4, 5)

| Material | Yield Stress (MPa) | Ultimate Stress (MPa) |
|---|---|---|
| Stainless steel | 700 | 850 |
| Cobalt alloy | 490 | 700 |
| Titanium alloy | 1100 | 1250 |
| Bone tissue | 85 | 120 |
| PMMA | — | 35 |
| UHMWPE | 14 | 27 |
| Patellar ligament | — | 58 |

stress different from the other two metals. For a material like stainless steel, the ultimate stress is only slightly higher than the yield stress. The ultimate strain, however, is several thousand times higher than the yield strain. Contrast this with cortical bone tissue (Fig. 4.18), for which the ultimate strain is only several times higher than the yield strain. Such distinctions become important in the choice of materials for particular applications. In applications where overloads cannot be allowed to produce rupture, a material with a high value of ultimate strain must be chosen. Because of the importance of this concept, a property has been defined that is useful in characterizing the amount of strain that can be tolerated before rupture. *The property of ductility is the strain at rupture (ultimate strain) in a material that undergoes inelastic deformation.* The ductility of bone is 3 percent, of 316L stainless steel is 30 percent, and of UHMWPE is 300 percent.

It is important to distinguish the concepts of elastic deformation and brittle behavior from those of inelastic deformation and ductile behavior. Both PMMA and rubber are brittle, elastic materials. Under tensile loading, both fail by brittle fracture, although the rubber clearly suffers a much larger elastic deformation. Thus, brittle failure is not limited to materials of high elastic modulus (low deformation to failure), but also encompasses materials of low elastic modulus (high deformation to failure). Contrast this with the stress-versus-strain curves for bone tissue and stainless steel, both ductile materials (Fig. 4.18). Bone exhibits about the same strain to failure as PMMA, a brittle material, and stainless steel exhibits considerably more strain to failure than either of these two materials.

Whereas the elastic modulus of stainless steel cannot be appreciably altered by mechanical or thermal treatments, other properties—specifically, ductility and yield stress—can be modified by such treatments. One common method used to make stainless steel "stronger" is to cold-work the material. This involves either squeezing the material between rollers to reduce its cross-sectional size or drawing the material through a series of dies to achieve the same result. Both methods are performed at temperatures well below the melting point of the steel (hence the term *cold work*).

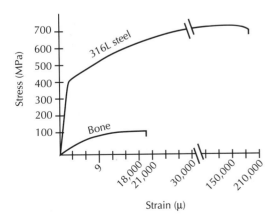

**Figure 4.18.**    Stress-versus-strain curves for bone tissue and stainless steel show that both are ductile materials, though the steel has a much higher ductility.

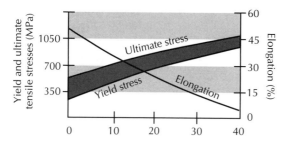

**Figure 4.19.** For 316L stainless steel with increased cold-working, the yield and ultimate tensile stress increases while the ductility decreases (6).

When stainless steel is worked in this manner, the microstructure of the material is altered and the grain size (the average size of the metallic crystals within the material) is reduced. These structural changes have two primary effects, namely, increasing the yield stress and decreasing the ductility (Fig. 4.19). We can achieve appreciable gains in yield stress while maintaining sufficient ductility for most practical orthopaedic applications. In fact, most of the stainless steel used for orthopaedic applications has had its ductility reduced to about 30 percent with an associated doubling of the yield stress.

## CYCLIC LOAD BEHAVIOR

In seeking answers to questions concerning trauma or situations of maximum tolerable loads, we rely on the static ultimate properties of the materials. Not all situations of interest, however, involve single (one-time) loading. In many instances repeated loads are the usual pattern. Is the resistance to failure of a structure or the materials composing the structure different when the loads are applied repeatedly as compared with a single load application? The answer is a resounding yes! We must therefore examine the way materials respond to repeated (cyclic) loads.

To determine the ultimate properties of bone tissue under compressive loading, we simply loaded the material until we observed gross rupture of the specimen. Cyclic testing to determine the failure properties is not as simple. For example, if bone tissue is loaded to 90 percent of the tensile yield stress, the material shows no appreciable damage during the first loading cycle. This is to be expected, since the yield stress is not exceeded. However, after continued cyclic loading through 350 cycles, the specimen will exhibit a significantly decreased elastic modulus (Fig. 4.20). If the experiment is repeated at a slightly lower stress, the specimen is able to withstand many more cycles before exhibiting a similar change in elastic behavior. In both cases, examination of the specimen will reveal microstructural damage to the bone tissue.

This type of test establishes two important concepts with respect to the ability of bone tissue to withstand cyclic loads. The first is that cyclic loading produces microstructural damage that accumulates with each loading cycle. The second concept is that the damage accumulates faster at higher intensities of cyclic loading. A similar pattern is seen in metallic materials. When stainless steel is cyclically loaded with sufficient intensity for a sufficient number of loading cycles, cracks tend to initiate and grow in the material. Such cracks can be seen in the stem portion of the femoral component of a total hip replacement (Fig. 4.21). *This complex failure response to cyclic loading is termed fatigue failure.*

If we cyclically load a specimen of stainless steel with a tensile load that maintains a stress level in the material equal to 80 percent of the yield stress, we observe no appreciable change in either the mechanical behavior or the

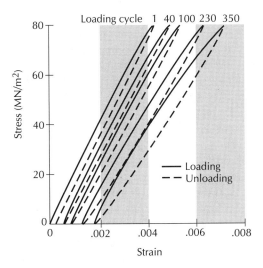

**Figure 4.20.** When bone tissue is loaded cyclically to 90 percent of its tensile yield strength, nonreversible behavior (damage) is seen. By the 350th loading cycle, the elastic modulus has changed appreciably (7).

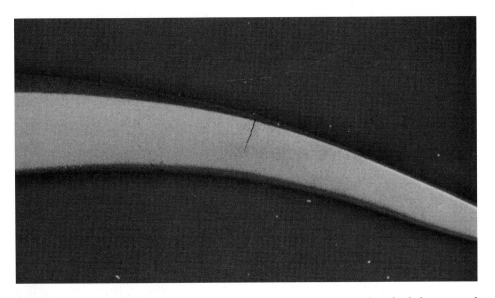

**Figure 4.21.** Cyclic loading led to the growth of the fatigue crack, which has caused almost complete fracture of this hip stem.

appearance of the specimen for about a million cycles of loading. However, careful observation during the next 100,000 cycles of loading reveals the initiation of microscopically small cracks on the surface of the specimen. Although the specimen now contains cracks, because of their very small size, no appreciable change in the mechanical behavior is yet noted. As we continue to load the steel specimen through the next several hundred thousand cycles, we observe an increase in the size of at least one of the cracks. As this crack penetrates deeper into the material, small changes in the loading response of the specimen are noted. Because of the crack, there is less cross-sectional area to resist the applied load, so the specimen's stiffness decreases. Also, the stress increases in the remaining material at the end of the crack.

As the load is repeated for the next few hundred cycles, the crack grows more rapidly. At some point, the remaining cross-sectional area of the specimen can no longer sustain the applied load, and the specimen ruptures. While the crack is growing, we do not notice any shape change or ductile behavior of the specimen. When the specimen finally ruptures, there is some associated shape change in the immediate vicinity of final rupture.

This type of experiment teaches important lessons about fatigue failure. One lesson is that a large portion of the cyclic loading history (typically, about the first 80 percent) is associated with initiating fatigue cracks. Subsequent propagation of one crack up to the rupture point requires far fewer loading cycles. Thus, any factor that encourages initiation of a crack will have a disastrous consequence on the fatigue life of a structure. In the simplest example, if one were to cut the surface of the test specimen with a scalpel, the resulting "scratch" would be virtually indistinguishable from a crack initiated after a million cycles. Thus, in this simple tension test, we could decrease the fatigue life (the number of cycles to failure) by 80 percent by scratching the surface of the specimen.

Another lesson that this type of experiment teaches us about fatigue is that there is a strong negative correlation between the intensity of loading and the number of loading cycles required for failure. Repeating the test at a load intensity necessary to maintain a stress level in the stainless steel equal to 70 percent of the yield stress will result in a cyclic life of many millions of cycles, considerably more than the 1 to 2 million cycles measured at 80 percent of yield stress. Lowering the cyclically applied stress further to 60 percent of the yield stress will result in a fatigue life of 10 million or more cycles.

In each case, the vast majority of the loading cycles are involved in initiating the crack. However, if we plot the number of cycles required for failure as a function of the stress intensity, we observe a strong, nonlinear relationship. If we replot the cycles data on a logarithmic scale, we observe an approximately linear inverse relationship with the applied stress, until the stress reaches about 60 percent of the yield stress. Such a plot is shown for cobalt alloy in Figure 4.22. Testing specimens at lower stresses does not induce fatigue failure, even at 100 million cycles. *We term this stress, below which fatigue cracks do not usually begin to form, the endurance limit or fatigue strength of the material.* Endurance limits for the common orthopaedic metallic alloys are given in Table 4.3.

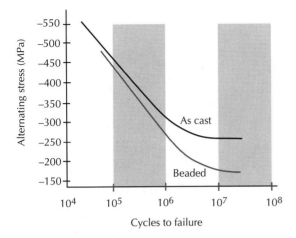

**Figure 4.22.** The plot depicting number of cycles to failure versus stress amplitude is shown for "as cast" cobalt alloy and cobalt alloy with a sintered, beaded surface (8). The specimens are exposed to reverse bending, subjecting them to alternating compression and tension stresses.

**Table 4.3.** Endurance Limits for Common Orthopaedic Metallic Alloys

| Material | Endurance Limit (MPa) |
|---|---|
| Stainless steel | 325 |
| Cobalt alloy | 330 |
| Titanium alloy | 525 |

It is obviously desirable to maintain the stresses induced in orthopaedic implants below the endurance limit. However, this is not always possible. Size and space restrictions, such as those in the medullary space of the femoral neck, preclude the designing of devices, such as nail-plates, with cross-sections large enough to guarantee against fatigue failure. Other geometric factors also contribute to the high stresses associated with fatigue failure. The screw hole in a bone plate, for example, causes an abrupt change in the plate's cross-section. This causes the strains and stresses adjacent to the hole to be greatly elevated over those in locations remote from the hole. This geometric effect, known as a *stress concentration*, usually results in local stresses that exceed the endurance limit of the plate material. It is a well-known clinical phenomenon that, in the presence of a nonunion, bone plates are at risk for fatigue failure after several months of implantation.

A stress concentration can result from any shape discontinuity and can affect orthopaedic implants in several subtle ways. We previously noted that a scratch on an implant can function as if it were a fatigue-initiated crack,

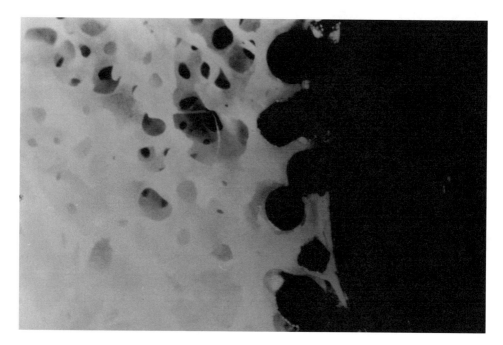

**Figure 4.23.** The cross-section of a test specimen used for Figure 4.22 would resemble the cross-section of this tibial component. Note the sharp notches formed by the surface and the attached beads.

dramatically reducing the fatigue life of the implant. Surface finishes (other than highly polished surfaces) can behave in a similar manner. Examine the photomicrograph in Figure 4.23 of a cross-section of a femoral stem on which a layer of beads has been sintered. The sintering process causes the metallic beads to fuse to the metallic substrate. Notice the sharp transition between the surface of the bead and the substrate. This geometric transition acts in much the same manner as the scalpel scratch in mimicking the shape of an initiated crack. Thus, coatings that introduce irregularities in a metallic surface can drastically reduce the fatigue life of the implant.

## *References*

1. Reilly DT, Burstein AH. The elastic and ultimate properties of compact bone tissue. J Biomech 1975;8:393-405.
2. Robinson RP, Wright TM, Burstein AH. The mechanical properties of polymethylmethacrylate bone cements. J Biomed Mater Res 1981;15:203-208.
3. Wright TM, Rimnac CM. Ultra high molecular weight polyethylene. In: Morrey B, ed. Joint replacement arthroplasty. New York: Churchill Livingstone, 1991:37-45.
4. Wright TM, Burstein AH. Musculoskeletal biomechanics. In: Evarts CM, ed. Surgery of the musculoskeletal system, 2nd ed. New York: Churchill Livingstone, 1990:231-271.

5. Noyes FR, Butler DL, Grood ES, Zernicke RF, Hefzy MS. Biomechanical analysis of human ligament grafts used in knee-ligament repairs and reconstructions. J Bone Joint Surg 1984;66A:344-352.
6. Lyman T, ed. Metals handbook, Vol. 1. Properties and selection of metals. 8th ed. Metals Park, Ohio: American Society for Metals, 1961:544.
7. Carter DR, Hayes WC. Compact bone fatigue damage, I. Residual strength and stiffness. J Biomech 1977;10:325-337.
8. Georgette FS, Davidson JA. The effect of HIPing on the fatigue and tensile strength of a cast, porous-coated Co-Cr-Mo alloy. J Biomed Mater Res 1986;20:1229-1248.

**5**

# MECHANICAL BEHAVIOR
# OF SKELETAL STRUCTURES

**AXIAL LOAD**
**BENDING LOAD**
**TORSIONAL LOAD**

In Chapter 1 we developed methods to examine the loads imposed on skeletal structures. We created free-body diagrams and used the laws of equilibrium to establish the forces and moments acting on various skeletal structures. In Chapter 4 we developed definitions of material properties that allow us to characterize and quantify a material's response to imposed loads. We will now combine these two concepts to examine the mechanical behavior of skeletal structures. Our goal is to determine whether a particular structure is capable of performing appropriately in its loaded environment. Will the structure maintain its shape? Will it break? If it is an implant, will it unduly influence its host structure?

In examining the mechanical behavior of a structure, we must analyze the structure in its entirety. Our concept or definition of a particular structure is of paramount importance. As with our analysis of a free body, all forces and moments acting on the structure will influence its mechanical behavior. Therefore, we will be careful and thorough in delineating the structure of interest.

Structures are categorized neither according to their shape and size nor according to the materials of which they are composed. Instead, structures are categorized according to the type of load to which they are subjected. We will detail the behavior of structures subjected to axial load, bending load, and torsional load. Structures with distributed loads and shared loads will be briefly described, and examples for further study will be identified.

## AXIAL LOAD

The simplest loading situation that a structure can experience is an axial load. To illustrate this concept, we will examine the patellar ligament in a subject rising from a chair, a situation we introduced in Chapter 1. We wish to ask several questions. What is the magnitude of the load applied to the ligament? What is the intensity of the stress within the fibers of the ligament? Can a portion of the ligament be safely used as a donor site for ligament transplant?

For this analysis, we will define the patellar ligament as that structure comprising the soft tissue attachments between the patella and the tibia, as well as the bony tissue into which the ligamentous fibers penetrate. As a loading situation, we will reconsider Figure 1.14, which shows the lower limb of a subject rising from a chair. As we noted in Chapter 1, ligamentous structures will support only loads that tend to pull the ligamentous fibers in the direction of their axis. *This loading situation is termed tensile axial loading.* In the case of a ligament whose fibers are essentially parallel and of the same length, it is reasonable to assume that all the fibers in the ligament cross-section share the load. For some ligamentous structures, such as the cruciate ligaments of the knee, whose fiber bundles are not parallel, imposed loads are not shared equally among all the fibers.

Let's examine the patellar ligament with regard to its ability to maintain its shape and to resist rupture under the imposed load. Our free-body analysis of the knee in Chapter 1 showed that the imposed load that the ligament must carry is 410 newtons. While this is a considerable load, it does not represent an extreme load, since the subject was using both legs to rise from the chair and was assisting this activity with some support from the arms of the chair.

Under this load, how much distortion is imposed on the ligament? We may either calculate the distortion based on the size of the ligament, its material properties, and the imposed load, or we may measure the distortion in an appropriate experiment. Consider the first method. We have observed that a structure under axial load elongates because the material elastically deforms. The amount of elongation that each unit length of the material undergoes is equal to the stress intensity divided by the elastic modulus $(E)$. The stress intensity was shown in Equation 4.1 to be the force $(F)$ divided by the cross-sectional area $(A)$. Therefore, the unit elongation in the structure is

$$\text{Unit elongation} = \frac{F}{A \times E} \tag{5.1}$$

Since each unit length of the structure contributes this amount of elongation, the entire structure will elongate an amount equal to the length $(L)$ of the structure multiplied by the unit elongation (as determined from Equation 5.1):

$$\text{Elongation} = \frac{F \times L}{A \times E} \tag{5.2}$$

We have noted that the patellar ligament is reasonably constant in cross-sectional area throughout its length. For structures with varying cross-sectional area, calculation of the total elongation is more cumbersome in that it requires a summation of the elongations of the unit lengths.

For the patellar ligament, the length is 0.03 meters, the cross-sectional area is 74 square millimeters, and the elastic modulus is 400 megapascals. Substituting these values, together with the 410-newton applied force, into Equation 5.2, the total elongation is

$$\text{Elongation} = \frac{410 \text{ N} \times 0.03 \text{ m}}{400 \text{ MPa} \times 0.000074 \text{ m}^2}$$

$$= 0.0004 \text{ m}$$

This elongation represents only the elongation of the ligament fibers. It does not represent elongation of the bony ends of the ligament.

If the experimental method is used to determine ligament elongation, the result will be somewhat greater than the analytical result, since in most test methodologies the ligament is held by its bony attachments to measure total elongation between the holding points. This typifies a common dilemma in determining structural distortion due to applied loads. The analytical technique considers an idealized structure, whereas the experimental technique uses attachment points for load application that can themselves contribute to the overall measured distortion.

## Axial Stiffness

We can now define the structural stiffness of the patellar ligament from both analytical and experimental results. *Structural stiffness is the ratio of the applied load (force or moment) to the resulting distortion (displacement or rotation)*:

$$\text{Structural stiffness} = \frac{\text{Applied load}}{\text{Resulting distortion}} \qquad (5.3)$$

By substituting for the unit elongation from Equation 5.1 into Equation 5.2, we can see that the structural stiffness of the ligament under axial load is

$$\text{Structural stiffness} = \frac{E \times A}{L} \qquad (5.4)$$

In the case of the ligament, the analytical structural stiffness is (from Equation 5.4)

$$\text{Structural stiffness}_{\text{Pat Lig}} = \frac{400 \text{ MPa} \times 0.000074 \text{ m}^2}{0.03 \text{ m}}$$

$$= 987{,}000 \text{ N/m}$$

The experimentally measured stiffness is about 503,000 newtons/meter [1]. We expect this value to be lower than the analytical result because of the effects of attachment point distortion in the grips and the contribution from the bony ends to total elongation.

Structural stiffness reflects the ability of a structure to maintain its shape while under load. If we had only the experimentally measured stiffness, we could calculate the amount of elongation developed in the patellar ligament (from Equation 5.3):

$$\text{Elongation} = \frac{\text{Load}}{\text{Structural stiffness}}$$

$$= \frac{410 \text{ N}}{503{,}000 \text{ N/m}}$$

$$= 0.0008 \text{ m}$$

Thus, the patellar ligament elongates less than 1 millimeter when our subject rises from the chair. This small elongation allows maintenance of the essential geometry of the patellofemoral joint. Note that structural stiffness is dependent upon both the size and shape of the structure (length and cross-sectional area for the case of axial loading), as well as the material properties of the ligament tissue (elastic modulus for the case of axial loading). These two factors are otherwise independent, since the size and shape of a structure does not depend on any material property. Thus, structural stiffness can be altered either by changes in the geometry of the structure or changes in the elastic modulus of the structure's material.

What, then, will be the effect on the structural stiffness of the remaining patellar ligament if one-third of the ligament is removed to be used as a graft? The removal will result in a decrease in the cross-sectional area of the ligament to two-thirds its original area, and, as can be seen from Equation 5.4, the structural stiffness will be two-thirds that of the original ligament. In removing the middle third of the ligament, we have not altered the length of the remaining ligament or the elastic modulus of the remaining ligamentous material.

The reduction in structural stiffness caused by removing the middle third of the ligament will result in an increase of the structural deformation of the ligament when the subject rises from the chair. The axial load of 410 newtons will produce an elongation one and one-half times the elongation in the original ligament. Whether this 50 percent increase in elongation (to almost 1½ millimeters) will have observable clinical consequences is not known.

### Axial Strength

Let's return to the question that must be in the mind of the orthopaedic surgeon when he or she removes the middle third of the patellar ligament: Will the remaining ligament rupture under load? To answer this question, we will calculate the stress intensity in the ligamentous material for both the natural and altered conditions. The stress intensity in the material of a structure with a uniform cross-section subjected to a tensile axial load is equal to the load divided by the cross-sectional area (Equation 4.1). For the natural patellar ligament, the stress is

$$\text{Stress} = \frac{410 \text{ N}}{0.000074 \text{ m}^2}$$

$$= 5.5 \text{ MPa}$$

Notice that this stress is well below the 58-megapascal stress required for the rupture of normal patellar ligament tissue (Table 4.2).

After one-third of the patellar ligament is removed for use as a graft, the cross-sectional area is reduced to 49 square millimeters, and the stress in the remaining ligamentous material increases by 50 percent, to 8.25 megapascals. This is still well below the rupture strength of the material. Remember, however, that in this example our subject distributed the load between both legs when rising from the chair. In more strenuous, single-legged activities such as stair climbing, where patellar ligament loads may approach three times body weight, stresses in the remaining material of the patellar ligament might approach the rupture stress:

$$\text{Stress} = \frac{3 \times \text{Body weight}}{\text{Area}}$$

$$= 42.3 \text{ MPa}$$

We generally describe the strength of a structure by the maximum load that the structure can withstand before material failure. In the case of the patellar ligament, the load that would cause failure can be found directly from Equation 4.1. If we solve this equation for the load required to produce a rupture stress, we find that the rupture load is

$$\text{Rupture load} = \text{Ultimate stress} \times \text{Area}$$

$$= 58 \text{ MPa} \times 0.000074 \text{ m}^2$$

$$= 4292 \text{ N}$$

Like structural stiffness, structural strength is dependent upon a geometric property of the structure and a material property. For structures subjected to axial loads, the geometric property that contributes to strength is the cross-sectional area. The material property that determines strength is the rupture (ultimate) stress.

## BENDING LOAD

We have examined structures of simple shape subjected to axial load. Now let's examine a simple structure that must carry loads perpendicular to its long axis. An example of this type of structure is a bone plate (Fig. 5.1). Let's imagine that the bone has external loads that tend to put the femur in a varus position and that, because of the unstable nature of the fracture, all the loads transmitted between the proximal and distal bone fragments must be carried by the plate.

### Moment Distribution

The actual loads on the plate are shown in Figure 5.2A. If we replace the actual loads with four idealized forces, a free body of the plate would consist of loads at either end of the plate caused by the tension in the screws and loads near the fracture site caused by contact with the bone (Fig. 5.2B). We wish to determine the stresses in the bone plate so that we may investigate both the distortion of the plate and the likelihood of its rupture. We begin by determining the forces that act within the confines of the plate.

During a normal walking cycle, a 90-newton-meter moment may be created on the femur (Fig. 5.1). In a manner similar to our process in examining the tendon (Fig. 4.3), we will examine a portion of the plate and use the laws of equilibrium to determine the forces and moments acting across its internal surfaces.

We will first examine the proximal half of the plate (Fig. 5.3). A free-body analysis considering only the 90-newton-meter bending moment shows the two idealized forces to be 1500 newtons each. We will next examine a segment of the proximal portion of the plate (Fig. 5.4). For our purposes, we will consider the plate to be rectangular in cross-section. The section at the imaginary cut can generally be expected to have both a force and a moment acting on its surface. The source of the force and moment is, of course, the

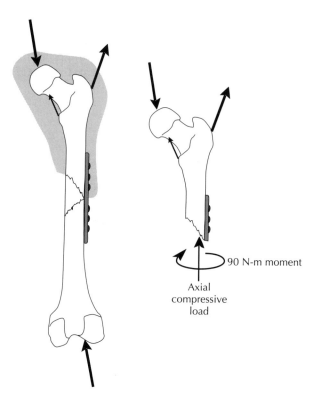

**Figure 5.1.** A bone plate applied to the femur will experience bending loads as a result of the muscle and joint reaction loads acting on the femur. The free-body analysis of the proximal portion shows the plate resisting a 90-newton-meter bending moment, together with an axial compressive load.

**Figure 5.2.** *A.* A free-body diagram of the bone plate from Figure 5.1 includes loads caused by tension in the screws and loads caused by contact with the bone. *B.* The load distribution on the plate can be idealized as a four-point bending load (two loads from the screws and two loads from contact with the bone).

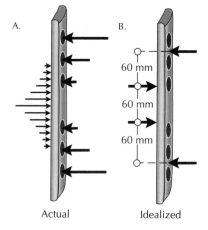

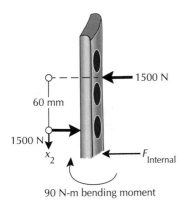

**Figure 5.3.** A free-body diagram of the proximal portion of the plate reveals that 1500 newtons of load are required to maintain force and moment equilibrium.

60 mm

1500 N

1500 N

$x_2$

$F_{Internal}$

90 N-m bending moment

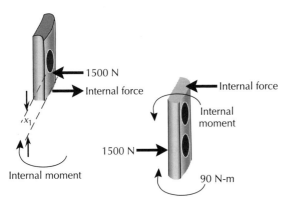

1500 N

Internal force

Internal force

Internal moment

1500 N

$x_1$

Internal moment

Internal moment

90 N-m

**Figure 5.4.** A free-body analysis of a segment of the proximal portion (Fig. 5.3) reveals an internal moment and an internal force that maintain the segment in equilibrium.

molecular forces across the contiguous surface of the plate. If we were to examine the distal segment of the proximal portion, we would recognize that its proximal surface contains a force and a moment of equal intensity but opposite direction to that contained on the distal surface of the proximal segment (Fig. 5.4).

Because these forces and moments are created by reaction of one internal surface against another internal surface, they are called internal forces and internal moments. This distinguishes them from forces and moments applied externally to the plate. Applying the law of equilibrium stating that the sum of the forces on the proximal segment of the plate must total zero (Equation 1.3),

$$\sum \text{Forces}_{\text{Horizontal}} = 1500 \text{ N} + F_{\text{Internal}} = 0$$

$$F_{\text{Internal}} = -1500 \text{ N}$$

Similarly, applying the law of equilibrium that states that the sum of the moments on the proximal segment of the plate must total zero (Equation 1.4),

$$\sum \text{Moments} = 1500 \text{ N} \times x_1 \text{ m} + M_{\text{Internal}} = 0$$

$$M_{\text{Internal}} = -1500 \times x_1 \text{ N} \cdot \text{m}$$

where $x_1$ is the distance from the 1500-newton external load to the imaginary cut section. This calculation shows that the amount of internal moment at any cross-section in the proximal segment of the plate depends upon the location of the cross-section. This is in contrast to the internal transverse force, whose magnitude does not depend upon the distance $x_1$. Thus, a shear force of 1500 newtons will exist at every cross-section in the proximal segment.

To illustrate, if we examine the cross-section for which $x_1$ equals 0.01 meters, the internal moment will be 15 newton-meters. If we choose the largest possible value of $x_1$ (0.06 meters), the internal moment will be 90 newton-meters. Therefore, we can see that the internal moment in the proximal segment of the bone plate varies from zero where the screw load is applied to a maximum of 90 newton-meters at the point of application of the bone contact force. The transverse force, however, is constant over this portion of the plate. In a similar manner, forces and moments in the distal segment will be a reflection of those in the proximal segment.

If we wish to find the internal moment in the central portion of the plate, we can return to the free body shown in Figure 5.3. Note that this free body includes both a proximal force provided by the bone screw and a central force provided by contact with the bone. Using Equation 1.3 for the force in the horizontal direction, we can determine the value of the internal transverse force on the central portion of the plate:

$$\sum \text{Forces} = 1500 \text{ N} - 1500 \text{ N} + F_{\text{Internal}}$$

$$F_{\text{Internal}} = 0$$

Note that equilibrium does not require any internal transverse force at this location. The sum of the two externally applied loads on the free body is zero.

Moment equilibrium (Equation 1.4) shows that the internal moment is

$$\sum \text{Moments} = 1500 \text{ N} \times x_2 \text{ m} - 1500 \text{ N} \times (0.06 + x_2) \text{ m} + M_{\text{internal}} = 0$$

$$M_{\text{internal}} = 90 \text{ N} \cdot \text{m}$$

Note that the internal moment does not depend upon the distance, $x_2$. Therefore, any cross-section located between the two central loads on the bone plate will have the same 90-newton-meter internal moment.

The situation that exists from either tip of the bone plate to either of the central loads is known as a *linearly varying bending moment* or a *cantilever* (that is, support at one end with a load applied at the tip). The situation that exists in the central portion of the plate is termed *constant moment* or *pure bending*. This term implies that there is only an internal moment and no internal transverse force.

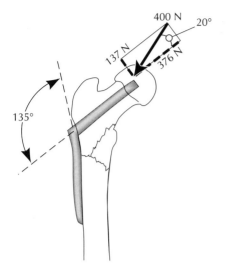

**Figure 5.5.** A nail-plate used to fix an intertrochanteric fracture is loaded to 400 N. The components of the applied load parallel and perpendicular to the axis of the nail are shown.

## Combined Loads

Many situations arise in which the applied loads on a structure are neither axially nor transversely oriented. Consider the nail-plate in Figure 5.5 that is used to fix an unstable intertrochanteric fracture. Let's assume that, in a static standing posture, the femoral head must support a load of 400 newtons acting at an angle of 20 degrees relative to the axis of the nail. Because of the instability at the fracture site, the bone fragments may not be able to carry any of this load initially. Instead, the nail-plate may be required to support the entire load.

Even though the load is oriented neither parallel nor perpendicular to the axis of the nail, we can examine the situation by resolving the applied external force into two components, one parallel and one perpendicular to the nail axis. The component parallel to the axis causes a compressive load on the nail. This component will be:

$$\text{Force}_{\parallel} = 400 \text{ N} \times \cos 20°$$
$$= 376 \text{ N}$$

The component perpendicular to the axis creates a bending moment. This component will be:

$$\text{Force}_{\perp} = 400 \text{ N} \times \sin 20°$$
$$= 137 \text{ N}$$

In determining the amount of distortion, as well as the tendency for the nail to rupture, we can analyze each of the two loading situations separately and then combine the results.

The axial loading situation is similar to that described previously for the patellar ligament. The only conceptual difference is that compressive stresses and shortening are the results of the 376-newton compressive load component on the nail, as compared to the tensile stresses and elongation that occurred as a result of the tensile load on the ligament.

Let's examine the internal forces and moments produced by the transverse component of the load. We will create a free body of the proximal portion of the nail-plate (Fig. 5.6) and apply the laws of equilibrium. From force equilibrium in the transverse direction (Equation 1.3), we see that the internal force that exists at section $A$ must be equal to the transverse component of the applied load:

$$\sum \text{Forces} = 137 \text{ N} - F_{\text{Internal}} = 0$$

$$F_{\text{Internal}} = 137 \text{ N}$$

Applying moment equilibrium (Equation 1.4) demonstrates that the internal moment must be equal to the transverse component of the external load multiplied by the distance, $x$, from the tip of the nail to section $A$:

$$\sum \text{Moments} = 137 \text{ N} \times x \text{ m} - M_{\text{Internal}} = 0$$

$$M_{\text{Internal}} = 137 \times x \text{ N} \cdot \text{m}$$

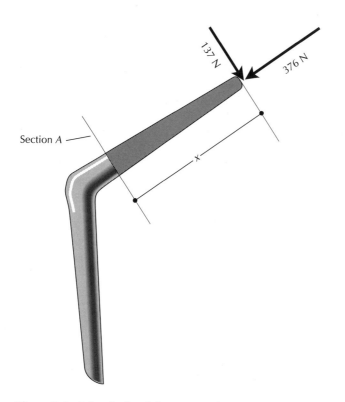

**Figure 5.6.** A free body of the proximal portion of the nail can be used to show that the internal moment varies linearly with the distance, $x$, from the tip of the nail.

Thus, the nail portion of the nail-plate is a cantilever beam with a linearly varying internal bending moment.

## Stress Distribution

Let's return to our previous example and ask how much load (force and moment) can be applied to the plate before a condition will exist that makes the plate unsatisfactory for its intended function. There are two conditions encountered clinically that cause the plate to cease to function satisfactorily. The first condition is permanent (or plastic) deformation of the plate. This condition arises when the plate is loaded with sufficient intensity to surpass the material's yield stress. Since bone plates are usually made from 316L stainless steel, if the stress exceeds 700 megapascals (Table 4.2), the plate will permanently deform and angulate the femur at the fracture site, inhibiting proper healing.

The second condition that will inhibit bony union is rupture of the plate by the fatigue process. As described in Chapter 4, this would occur if enough load cycles of sufficient intensity were applied to cause a crack to initiate and propagate across the bone plate. This could occur if the stress intensity exceeded the fatigue strength of the stainless steel material (325 megapascals, from Table 4.3), and a sufficient time passed to accumulate the required number (10 million) of loading cycles.

Both of these failure conditions require a specific intensity of induced stress. How do we determine the stress induced in the bone plate under the influence of external transverse or bending loads? To develop an empirically based understanding of the types of stresses induced in a structure because of external transverse loading, let's consider the following experiment. We take a long, rectangular piece of rubber and inscribe longitudinal and transverse lines on its surface (Fig. 5.7A). We apply loads to this rubber "beam" similar to those applied to the plate (Fig. 5.2B). In the loaded condition, the lines on the surface of the beam no longer form a rectangular grid. The longitudinal lines are curved, whereas the transverse lines, while still essentially straight, are no longer parallel.

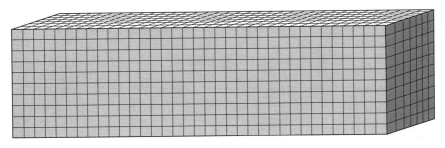

**Figure 5.7A.** A rubber beam with a rectangular cross-section has been inscribed with longitudinal and transverse lines.

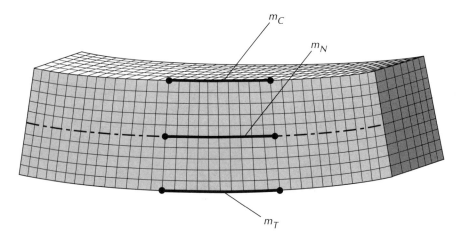

**Figure 5.7B.** Under the influence of the four loads, the longitudinal lines curve and the transverse lines are no longer parallel.

Let's examine the lengths of the segments of the longitudinal lines enclosed within the transverse lines. Typical among these are line segments $m_T$, $m_C$, and $m_N$ (Fig. 5.7B). Careful observations before and after loading will reveal no apparent change in the length of line segment $m_N$. Since this line segment, which happens to overlie the midline of the beam, has no length change, it is subject to no tensile or compressive strain. We can deduce that the midline of the beam experiences neither tensile nor compressive stress.

Contrast this with the case for line segment $m_T$, which in the loaded state is longer than it was in the unloaded condition. This elongation corresponds to a tensile strain, which implies a tensile stress on the transverse surfaces on this side of the beam. Similar observation of line segment $m_C$ reveals a shortening under load, corresponding to a compressive strain and an associated implication of compressive stress.

Further observation of the beam in the loaded condition reveals that all the longitudinal line segments on the same side of the midline have similar states of elongation. Thus, all the lines between $m_N$ and $m_C$ are shortened, and all the lines between $m_N$ and $m_T$ are elongated. We further note that because transverse lines have remained as straight lines under load, the amount of shortening or elongation of any particular longitudinal line segment is proportional to its location between the midline axis and the outer surface of the beam. Thus, if the line segment $m_{C1}$ (Fig. 5.7C) has decreased in length by an amount equal to $\Delta C$, line segment $m_{C2}$ will have decreased in length by $2\Delta C$, since it is twice the distance from the midline axis as segment $m_{C1}$. There is a similar proportionality in the amount of elongation of each of the longitudinal line segments in the region between $m_N$ and $m_T$.

The pattern of stresses (Fig. 5.8) implied by this observed deformation pattern is a linear distribution. *The central portion of the cross-section of the beam*

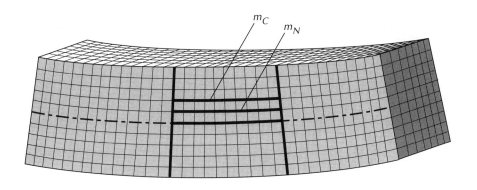

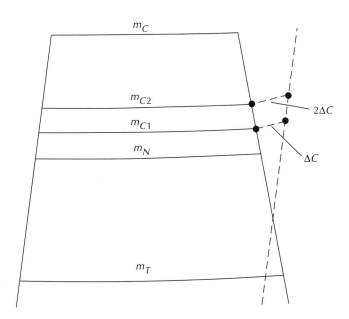

**Figure 5.7C.** The shortening of a line segment above the midline axis $(m_N)$ is proportional to its distance from the midline axis. Therefore, $m_{C2}$ shortens twice as much as $m_{C1}$, since it is twice as far from the midline.

*contains no stress. The portion that has no stress due to bending is often called the neutral axis.* The maximum stresses in both tension and compression are found at the outermost cross-sectional surface of the beam. At any particular section, the linear stress distribution will produce a particular force and a particular moment at the section of the beam. These forces and moments must, of course, correspond to the internal forces and internal moments acting on the beam.

**Figure 5.8.** The stress distribution in the bending of the rubber beam (Fig. 5.7) is linear across the beam with compressive stress in the top half, zero stress at the midline (the neutral axis), and tensile stress in the bottom half of the beam.

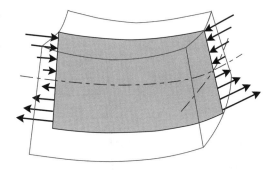

Let's first examine the net internal force that this stress distribution produces. Remembering that the force is equal to the stress multiplied by the cross-sectional area over which the stress acts, we can see that there would be no net force in the longitudinal direction. This is because stresses of the same magnitude but opposite directions (tension versus compression) act on surfaces that are symmetrically and equally distributed about the neutral axis. Thus, the tensile force produced on the surface bounded by $m_N$ and $m_T$ is equal in magnitude and opposite in direction to the compressive force acting on the surface bounded by $m_N$ and $m_C$. Since the cross-section of our "beam" at the free-body boundary (Fig. 5.7C) requires no net longitudinal force for equilibrium, our empirically derived stress distribution is suitable.

While the net internal force in the longitudinal direction produced by the linear stress distribution is zero, the same is not true of the net internal moment. To calculate the moment produced by the forces associated with the stresses, let's first calculate the net moment caused by the tensile and compressive forces acting on the two halves of the cross-section. To accomplish this, we will consider the cross-section as comprising many small area segments (Fig. 5.9). Each of these thin area segments may be thought of as having a uniform stress. We have already established that the stress on any area segment is proportional to the distance from the neutral axis. If the stress on the outermost area segment is denoted by $\sigma_{max}$ (the maximum normal stress), then the stress on every other area segment, $\sigma_x$, is equal to $\sigma_{max}$ multiplied by the ratio $x$ to $h/2$:

$$\sigma_x = \sigma_{max} \times \frac{x}{h/2}$$

We can now establish the force, $F_x$, on each of these area segments as

$$F_x = \text{Stress} \times \text{Area}$$
$$= \sigma_x \times \text{Area}$$
$$= \left(\sigma_{max} \times \frac{x}{h/2}\right) \times (b \times \Delta x)$$

Again, note that $\sigma_{max}$ is the particular maximum stress that must exist at the outermost area segment.

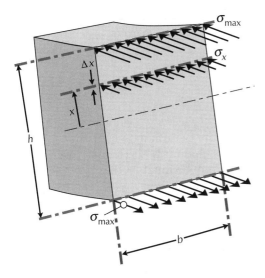

**Figure 5.9.** Each segment of area experiences a stress proportional to the distance, $x$, between the segment and the neutral axis.

We now must determine how much internal moment is produced by each of the forces acting on the area segments. If we consider the moments to be summed about the neutral axis, then the moment arm for each of the forces is equal to $x$ (Fig. 5.9). Thus, the moment, $M_x$, produced by the stress acting on an area segment that is a distance $x$ from the neutral axis is

$$M_x = \text{Force} \times \text{Moment arm}$$

$$= F_x \times x$$

$$= \left( \sigma_{max} \times \frac{x}{h/2} \times b \times \Delta x \right) \times x$$

The expression for $M_x$ can be rewritten as

$$M_x = \frac{\sigma_x}{h/2} \times (b \times \Delta x) \times x^2$$

To determine the total moment produced by all the area segments, their contributions must be added:

$$M_{Total} = \sum M_x$$

The result will be the sum of the area segments $(b \times \Delta x)$ multiplied by the square of the distance from the neutral axis $(x^2)$, multiplied by the maximum stress intensity $(\sigma_{max})$, and divided by the distance from the neutral axis to the outer surface $(h/2)$:

$$M_{Total} = \frac{\sigma_{max}}{h/2} \times \sum [(b \times \Delta x) \times x^2]$$

The term $[(b \times \Delta x) \times x^2]$ has a special meaning. *The property of a cross-section derived from adding together area segments multiplied by the square of the distance from the area segment to the neutral axis is known as the area moment of inertia, I, of the cross-section:*

$$I = \sum (b \times \Delta x) \times x^2 \qquad (5.5)$$

Note that the area segments farther from the neutral axis contribute significantly more to the area moment of inertia than area segments closer to the neutral axis, because their contribution is proportional to the *square* of their distances from the neutral axis. We may therefore rewrite our expression for the moment as

$$\text{Moment} = \sigma_{max} \times \frac{I}{(h/2)} \qquad (5.6)$$

Returning to the bone plate (Fig. 5.1), let's determine the stresses imposed on the plate if the patient is allowed only protected weight bearing. We will assume that, with protected weight bearing, the original applied loads (1500 newtons) are reduced by two-thirds, to 500 newtons. These loads would create a bending moment of 30 newton-meters. To determine the stress induced by this bending moment, we can rearrange Equation 5.6 and multiply the moment by the quantity $I/(h/2)$. For the plate, the area moment of inertia is calculated from the expression

$$I_{\text{Rectangle}} = \frac{b \times h^3}{12} \qquad (5.7)$$

which applies for all rectangular cross-sections with base dimension $b$ and height $h$.

For a bone plate with a base of 15 millimeters and a height of 4 millimeters, the area moment of inertia is (from Equation 5.7)

$$I_{\text{Plate}} = \frac{15 \text{ mm} \times (4 \text{ mm})^3}{12}$$

$$= 80 \text{ mm}^4$$

Since $h/2$ for the plate is 2 millimeters, the maximum stress induced at the surface of the plate due to the 30-newton-meter bending moment is

$$\sigma_{max} = M \times \frac{(h/2)}{I}$$

$$= 30 \text{ N} \cdot \text{m} \times \frac{2 \text{ mm}}{80 \text{ mm}^4}$$

$$= 750 \text{ MPa}$$

This is a rather high stress for type 316L stainless steel, given that the yield stress for this material is 700 megapascals (Table 4.2). This bone plate is severely stressed, even for modest bending loads on the femur. Thus, a bone plate cannot support even modest bending loads across an unstable fracture when the femur cannot share a portion of the bending moment.

We have now determined the stresses on a cross-section in the middle of the plate. We found from our free-body analysis that there will be no transverse force and a 30-newton-meter internal moment. Would the stress distribution at the cross-section be the same for the proximal section of the distal portion of the plate (Fig. 5.10)? Equilibrium conditions require a transverse force of 500 newtons on the cross-section at $A$ and an internal moment. In addition to the tensile and compressive stresses caused by this moment, we must have transverse (shear) stresses acting on the cross-section in response to the external 500-newton transverse load.

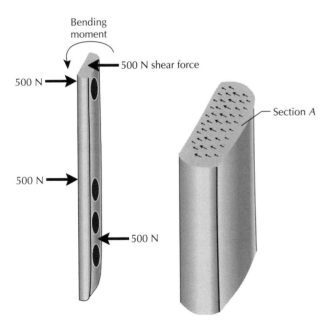

**Figure 5.10.** In the proximal section of the distal portion of the bone plate, near the externally applied 500-newton load, an internal shear force of 500 newtons is required to maintain equilibrium. The resulting shear stress distribution shows the maximum shear stress at the center of the cross-section.

The shear stress distribution that satisfies the equilibrium conditions is shown in Figure 5.10. Unlike the stresses induced by the internal bending moment, the shear stresses are maximum at the center of the cross-section and are zero at the surfaces of the cross-section. The magnitude of the maximum shear stress is quite low, only 15 megapascals. In most problems in orthopaedic biomechanics, the shear stresses induced in beams are quite low and are usually ignored.

What will be the stress in the plate if the plate is applied to the lateral surface of the femur, which is then exposed to the same 30-newton-meter bending moment? The plate will now be oriented so that its height dimension, $h$, is 15 millimeters and its base dimension, $b$, is 4 millimeters. This will change its area moment of inertia (Equation 5.7) to

$$I_{Plate} = \frac{4 \text{ mm} \times (15 \text{ mm})^3}{12}$$

$$= 1125 \text{ mm}^4$$

$h/2$ for the plate in this orientation will be 7.5 millimeters, and the resulting maximum stress at the outer surface of the plate will be

$$\sigma_{max} = 30 \text{ N} \cdot \text{m} \times \frac{7.5 \text{ mm}}{1125 \text{ mm}^4}$$

$$= 2000 \text{ MPa}$$

Thus, by changing the orientation of the plate so that its greatest dimension represents the thickness, we reduce the maximum stress by a factor of 3.75 compared with the stress when the smallest dimension represents the thickness. It must be realized in both cases that the bone has been assumed to carry no load. Good fracture fixation techniques require that, before a plate can be used, the fracture be "stabilized" to provide bony contact and load transmission across the fracture fragments. Without such stabilization, a single bone plate will be subjected to large stresses and will fail. Our example shows that this will occur even with protected weight bearing.

What bias is introduced by our assumption that the bone plate is rectangular? If we examine an actual cross-section of a bone plate, we see that it is not a simple rectangle. We cannot, therefore, use Equation 5.7 to calculate the area moment of inertia, since this expression is applicable only to rectangles. Instead, we must return to Equation 5.5. Carrying out the summation operation for the actual cross-section will give us the results shown in Table 5.1. Note that the cross-sectional properties of the actual bone plate are not grossly different from those of our rectangular plate.

### Bending Strength

We can now make an important observation about the bending strength of beams. *We define the strength of a beam as the largest bending moment that*

**Table 5.1.**  Area Moments of Inertia for Rectangle and for Bone Plate Cross-Sections

|  | $I_{\blacksquare}$ | $I_{\underline{\ }}$ |
|---|---|---|
| Rectangle | 1125 mm$^4$ | 80 mm$^4$ |
| Bone plate | 1068 mm$^4$ | 86 mm$^4$ |

*the beam can carry without causing the stress to exceed a critical limit.* This critical limit may be either the yield stress, if we don't want the beam to permanently deform; the ultimate stress, if we don't want the beam to rupture; or the endurance limit, if we don't want the beam to fracture in fatigue. Looking at Equation 5.6, we see that the strength of the beam is controlled by two factors. The first is the maximum tolerable stress, which of course, is a material property. The second factor is the area moment of inertia, $I$, of the cross-section divided by half the height, $h/2$. *This quantity, $I/(h/2)$, is often called the section modulus and is a property only of the size and shape of the beam's cross-section.* Therefore, in a situation analogous to our findings for tensile and compressive axial loading, the bending strength of a beam depends both upon a property of the material from which the structure is composed and upon a property of the geometry of the structure.

Let's examine the strength property of the cross-section in more detail. We have already seen that changing the orientation of the rectangular bone plate greatly alters the magnitude of the stress in the plate. The section modulus for the flat plate is

$$\text{Section modulus}_{\text{Flat}} = \frac{I}{h/2} = \frac{b \times h^2}{6}$$

$$= \frac{15 \text{ mm} \times (4 \text{ mm})^2}{6}$$

$$= 40 \text{ mm}^3$$

as compared with the section modulus for the plate positioned vertically with respect to the applied bending moment:

$$\text{Section modulus}_{\text{Vertical}} = \frac{4 \text{ mm} \times (15 \text{ mm})^2}{6}$$

$$= 150 \text{ mm}^3$$

Thus, by changing the geometry of the plate simply by changing its orientation with respect to the direction of the applied bending moment, the section modulus and hence the bending strength of the plate is increased by a factor of 3.75. Note that this is the same factor by which the maximum stress in the outer fiber was reduced by reorienting the plate (from 750 to 200 megapascals).

We can compare the strength property of this rectangular cross-section to the strength property of the stem portion of a long-stemmed femoral component for total hip replacement. Typically the stems are of approximately circular cross-section and are about 14 millimeters in diameter for adult patients. For a circular cross-section, $h/2$ is simply the radius, $r$, of the cross-section. The section modulus for the femoral stem can be calculated from the expression

$$\text{Section modulus} = \frac{I}{h/2} = \frac{(\pi \times r^4)/4}{r}$$

$$= \frac{\pi \times r^3}{4} \tag{5.8}$$

$$= 269 \text{ mm}^3$$

Thus, the 14-millimeter-diameter intramedullary stem, made from the same 316L stainless steel material as the bone plate, is 92 percent stronger than the plate when it is turned on edge.

Since the bending strength of a stem or rod varies as the cube of the radius of the rod, we can see the advantage of choosing the largest clinically acceptable diameter for an intramedullary rod for fracture fixation. The strength advantage gained in choosing an 11-millimeter-diameter rod over a 10-millimeter-diameter rod, for example, is the ratio of $11^3$ to $10^3$, or 1.33, for a 33 percent gain.

Not all intramedullary rods have a solid cross-section. Some rods have shapes that can be described as hollow cylinders. What will be the effect on the strength of a 14-millimeter intramedullary rod if we hollow the center to a 10-millimeter inner diameter? The strength of the hollow rod will be the section modulus for the solid 14-millimeter rod minus the section modulus for the 10-millimeter-diameter "inner rod" removed to make the hole. We have already determined the former to be 269 millimeters$^3$. The latter is 98 millimeters$^3$. The section modulus for the hollow rod is therefore 269 millimeters$^3$ minus 98 millimeters$^3$, or 171 millimeters$^3$. We have only 49 percent of the material remaining from the original solid rod after we make it hollow, but we have retained 64 percent of the bending strength. Hollow cylinders, therefore, are effective structures for resisting bending loads, because they possess high strength-to-weight ratios. They are not stronger than the same-diameter solid rod; they are merely lighter than a solid rod of the same strength. A solid rod of the same strength as the 14 millimeter hollow rod would be 12 millimeters in diameter and weigh $1\frac{1}{2}$ times as much.

We have now demonstrated two ways to control the bending strength of a beam. We can manipulate the shape of the beam to maximize its section modulus, or we can choose a material with appropriate strength properties.

## Composite Beams

We have shown that an unstable fracture (even with protected weight bearing) induces unacceptably large stresses in the bone plate. Let's examine the advantage of stabilizing the fracture with bone-to-bone contact across the fracture

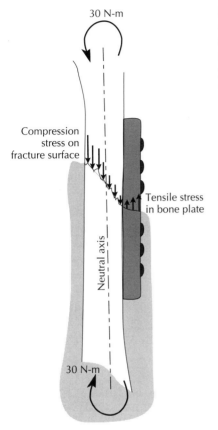

30 N-m

Compression
stress on
fracture surface

Tensile stress
in bone plate

Neutral axis

30 N-m

**Figure 5.11.** A plated long bone fracture un-der an external bending moment will act as a composite beam of metal and bone. The neutral axis exists somewhere within the bone near the plate. The stress distribution within the plate and the bone is shown.

site. After the fracture has been reduced, the surgeon applies the plate to that surface of the bone that is thought to carry the tensile stresses under normal cir-cumstances (Fig. 5.11). If the bone fragments are well reduced, the action of the applied external bending moment will elongate the plate, causing a small gap in the bone underneath the plate. At the same time, the bending moment will compress the cortex opposite the plate. A neutral axis will exist somewhere within the bone at an asymmetrical location near the plate (2). The strain, as in the previous example (Fig. 5.7), is still proportional to the distance from the neutral axis. However, a small strain in the metal, because of its relatively large elastic modulus, is associated with a larger stress as compared with the same strain in the bone tissue.

The overall effect, however, is to have a composite bone-metal beam whose cross-section is substantially larger than that of the plate alone. For the composite bone-plate structure, a 30-newton-meter bending moment will produce a 10-megapascal maximum compressive stress in the cortex and a 34-megapascal maximum tensile stress in the plate (3). This, of course, is a substantial reduction in the stress in the plate, and the stress in the bone is well within the stress tolerance of bone tissue (Table 4.2).

## Deflection of Beams

In examining orthopaedic implants to determine their suitability for a specific application, the surgeon must be concerned about the strength of the implant. There are additional considerations, however, that may be just as important. It is an accepted principle in fracture fixation that the displacement at the fracture site must be minimized. In most instances, this displacement is controlled by the structural stiffness of the fixation device. If we know the loads that the fixation device will carry, can we determine the deflection that will be induced at the fracture site? What must we know about the fixation device in order to calculate this deflection?

To answer these questions, consider again the example of a nail-plate used to fix an intertrochanteric fracture (Fig. 5.5). In the elderly patient, the most secure fit between the proximal femoral fragment and the hip nail is within the head of the femur. The proximal fragment will follow the nail if the nail deforms and hence will induce motion at the fracture site. As a relative measure of the motion induced at the fracture site, let's determine the deflection of the tip of the nail under physiological loading conditions.

For every beam subjected to bending loads, the deflection at any particular point on the beam is proportional to the bending moment multiplied by the square of the length of the beam:

$$\text{Deflection} \propto \text{Moment} \times \text{Length}^2$$

If the moment is caused by a load such as that acting on the tip of the nail (Fig. 5.5), then the magnitude of the moment is the force, $F$, multiplied by the length of the beam, $L$. For the case of a cantilevered nail,

$$\text{Deflection} \propto (F \times L) \times L^2$$
$$\propto F \times L^3$$

Two factors control the proportion between deflection and $F \times L^3$. One is a property of the material from which the beam is made. The other factor is a property of the cross-sectional shape of the beam. The material property that regulates deflection is the elastic modulus, $E$. The cross-sectional property is the area moment of inertia, $I$. For the cantilevered hip nail, the relationship between these variables and the deflection at the tip of the nail is given by the expression

$$\text{Deflection} = \frac{F \times L^3}{3 \times E \times I} \tag{5.9}$$

The numerical constant, 3, is associated with a cantilever beam. Other types of beams have other associated constants.

## Bending Rigidity

Our initial concern was the deflection at the tip of the nail. We define *the bending rigidity of the nail as the ratio between the applied load and the deflection at the tip of the nail*. Thus, if we know the bending rigidity, we can determine the total deflection by dividing the applied load by the rigidity. From Equation 5.9, we see that the bending rigidity (load/deflection) is

$$\text{Bending rigidity} = \frac{\text{Force}}{\text{Deflection}}$$

$$= \frac{3 \times E \times I}{L^3}$$

We see, therefore, that the bending rigidity is proportional to the elastic modulus multiplied by the area moment of inertia. In addition, for any cantilever beam, the rigidity will vary inversely with the cube of the beam's length.

It is often necessary to selectively design the rigidity of an orthopaedic implant. However, the choices of metallic materials for orthopaedic implants allow limited variation in elastic modulus (Table 4.1). The extreme range available is approximately 2 to 1, the ratio for cobalt alloy to titanium alloy. For a particular application, the length of the device is usually constrained by anatomy. It is therefore the cross-section of the device that provides the widest latitude of design choices.

Let's compute the deflection of a Jewett hip nail-plate. The nail is 86 millimeters long with an elastic modulus of 180 gigapascals (for stainless steel). The area moment of inertia for the Jewett nail is 19.5 millimeters$^4$ (4). Remembering from Figure 5.6 that the transverse load is 137 newtons, we can calculate the deflection at the tip of each nail (from Equation 5.9):

$$\text{Deflection}_{\text{Jewett}} = \frac{137 \text{ N} \times (86 \text{ mm})^3}{3 \times 180 \text{ GPa} \times 19.5 \text{ mm}^4}$$

$$= 8.3 \text{ mm}$$

This deflection could be quite meaningful in terms of the rate of union at the fracture site. The low rigidity of the Jewett nail-plate is an important factor in limiting the use of the device to stable fractures.

As a further example, let's reconsider our choice of either a 10-millimeter-diameter or an 11-millimeter-diameter intramedullary rod. What is the ratio of the bending rigidities of these rods? Of course, the ratio of the deflections at the fracture site will be the inverse of the ratio of the bending rigidities. If the rods are constructed from the same material (with the same elastic modulus), the comparative rigidities will be controlled by their area moments of inertia. For a solid circular cross-section, the area moment of inertia about a central bending axis is

$$I_{Circle} = \frac{\pi \times r^4}{4}$$  (5.10)

where $r$ is the radius of the circle. Therefore, the ratio of the bending rigidities of the two rods will be

$$\frac{Rigidity_{11}}{Rigidity_{10}} = \frac{I_{11}}{I_{10}} = \frac{r_{11}^4}{r_{10}^4} = \frac{Diameter_{11}^4}{Diameter_{10}^4} = \frac{11^4}{10^4}$$

$$= 1.46$$

Thus, the 11-millimeter intramedullary rod is 46 percent more rigid than the 10-millimeter rod. Since the deflection is inversely proportional to the rigidity, the 11-millimeter rod allows only 68 percent of the deflection of the 10-millimeter rod. It is interesting to note that our previous strength comparison of the two rods showed the larger rod to have a 33 percent advantage. This is because the bending strength of a beam with circular cross-section is proportional to the radius cubed (Equation 5.8), whereas its bending rigidity is proportional to the radius to the fourth power (Equation 5.10).

## Load-Deflection Behavior

Sometimes it is sufficient to know the elastic or reversible behavior of an implant structure, but there are often cases when permanent deformations are imposed, and patient care decisions must be made. As an example, consider the two-month follow-up "radiograph" shown in Figure 5.12. Measurement reveals that the tip of the nail has permanently deflected from its original, straight position by 4 millimeters. While this residual deflection produces a proximal fragment with an acceptable degree of varus, there are some serious implications for the healing process. The question we must ask is, what was the total deflection undergone by the nail tip, and consequently the proximal fragment, to result in the 4 millimeters of permanent deflection?

To answer this question, we will examine the history of the deformation during a loading cycle that allowed the residual deformation of 4 millimeters (Fig. 5.13). To produce the loading history, we simultaneously record load and deformation at the tip of the nail and plot one against the other. Both of these variables are plotted through the loading and unloading portions of the cycle. We note that the loading portion of the cycle has an initial straight-line region (to point A in Fig. 5.13). If the load is removed at any point in this initial loading phase, the unloading curve will be a straight line of the same slope overlying the loading curve. This is characteristic of fully reversible or elastic behavior (see Chapter 4). Removal of the load in this phase leaves no residual deformation, even with a maximum of 8 millimeters of deformation. We also observe that the slope of the curve in this straight-line region is change in force divided by change in deformation, which is our definition of bending rigidity.

When we increase the load above the last point in the linear region, we enter the nonlinear or plastic region. With such higher loads, the material suffers

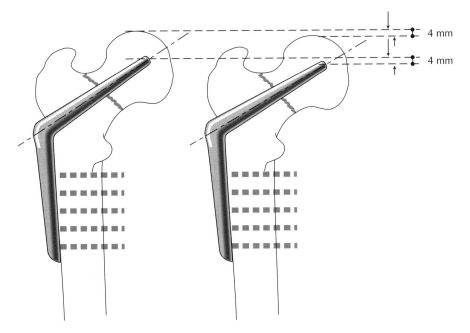

4 mm

4 mm

**Figure 5.12.** The postoperative radiograph shows a well-aligned, reduced fracture. The two-month follow-up radiograph, when superimposed over the original, shows 4 millimeters of "settling."

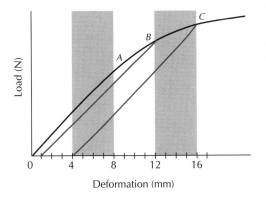

**Figure 5.13.** Load is plotted against deformation for a hip nail for both loading and unloading. Beyond point *A* residual deformation of the nail will remain after removal of the load.

stresses above the yield stress and hence permanently deforms. This results in permanent shape change in the hip nail. If we remove the load at point *B*, we note an essentially straight-line return parallel to the initial straight-line elastic portion of the loading curve. After unloading, there is a residual permanent deformation of 1 millimeter. Note that the maximum deformation at point *B* prior to unloading was 12 millimeters.

By judicious experimentation, we can arrive at loading point *C*. This is the point that produces a residual deformation of 4 millimeters. Thus, 4 millimeters of residual deformation required a total deformation of 16 millimeters. If we return to our clinical question, we can appreciate that the consequences of the 16-millimeter deformation are much more severe than is apparent from the residual deformation of 4 millimeters. The nail can safely undergo a deformation of up to 8 millimeters with no residual deformation, 12 millimeters with 1 millimeter of (hardly noticeable) deformation, and 16 millimeters with 4 millimeters of (very noticeable) deformation. Because surgeons seldom visualize the deformation of orthopaedic implants under the action of realistic physiological loads, they usually have a minimal intuitive sense of how large reversible deformations can be. The presence of even a small permanent deformation in an implant should be taken as an indication of a much larger total deformation.

A useful tool in evaluating the comparative performance of fracture fixation devices is a four-point bending test (Fig. 5.2). Implants are loaded beyond the point of reversible deformation, and a plot of bending (in the central segment) moment versus deformation is obtained. The methodology and geometry for testing orthopaedic implants has been standardized by the American Society for Testing and Materials (5, 6). The curves for bending moment versus deformation for tests on two intramedullary rods are shown in Figure 5.14, together with the bending moment curve for a femur. The rod size has been chosen so that these devices are appropriate fracture fixation implants for the femur. The characteristics of the three structures can be ascertained by close examination of the curves. We will first determine their relative rigidities. Similar to the rigidity of a load-versus-deformation test, the initial slope of the bending moment–versus–deformation curve is also a measure of the rigidity

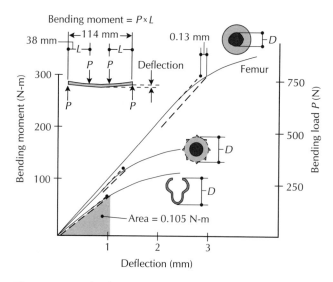

**Figure 5.14.** The four-point bending test results for two intramedullary rods and the matching femur show bending strength at the 0.13-millimeter offset (6). The energy required to produce bending failure is shown as the area under the curve of bending load (see right scale) versus deformation.

of the rod (see page 155). In this case, the hollow circular rod has a rigidity of $90 \times 10^3$ newton-meters/meter versus the hollow cloverleaf rod, which has a rigidity of $70 \times 10^3$ newton-meters/meter. The femur is more rigid than either rod ($100 \times 10^3$ newton-meters/meter).

The strength of the rod can be taken as the maximum bending moment that can be sustained before permanent deformation of the rod occurs. To determine the strength, we would like to observe the last point on the straight-line portion of the bending moment–versus–deformation curve. But there is no practical way to identify this point. A more repeatable, conventional method (6) is to draw a line parallel to the straight-line portion of the curve and off-set the line 0.13 millimeters (Fig. 5.14). *The bending strength of the rod is taken as the bending moment defined by the intersection of the offset line and the bending moment–versus–deformation curve.* For the hollow circular rod, the bending strength (125 newton-meters) is less than half that of the bone (300 newton-meters) but approximately 1.7 times that of the hollow cloverleaf rod (75 newton-meters). Because the circular rod and the bone are symmetrical shapes, their bending strengths and rigidities are the same for every direction of bending. The cloverleaf shape is not symmetrical; therefore, its properties will change depending on the direction of bending.

## Energy Absorption

Load-versus-deformation curves allow the calculation of the amount of energy that is stored in a beam during the loading cycle. When we wished to calculate strain energy in a bone plate, we calculated the area under the force-versus-extension curve (see Chapter 4, page 114). Since work is equal to force multiplied by the displacement through which the force moves, we can calculate work performed on the intramedullary rods and the femur in a similar manner. The product of force and displacement is again the area under the load-versus-deformation curve.

Let's compare the energy required to load the tested length (114 millimeters) of each structure to the point at which the material begins to plastically deform. Since this load defines the bending strength of each structure, we will be comparing the energies required to produce bending failure. For the hollow circular rod, 0.23 joules (newton-meters) of energy are required, slightly more than twice the 0.11 joules required for the cloverleaf rod (Fig. 5.14). The bone, however, requires 1.18 joules to induce plastic deformation. Thus, in terms of resistance to trauma, even a hollow circular rod that completely fills the medullary canal can absorb only one-fifth of the energy required to damage a bone.

Let's now compare the amounts of energy required to fracture the femur from a fall. At the instant of fracture of the femur, the area under the load-versus-deformation curve for the entire femur would be approximately 15 joules. Compare this with the 350 joules associated with a typical fall (Chapter 2, page 48). It is clear that the energy produced by a fall cannot be absorbed by one or even both femurs without causing a fracture. Since the intramedullary fixation rod has even less energy absorption capacity than the femur, these fixation devices will not protect against even modest, repeated trauma.

## TORSIONAL LOAD

The third common mode of loading is torsional load. Torsional loads produce moments, but unlike bending moments, torsional moments tend to twist structures such as bones. A typical example of torsional loading occurs in skiing. If a load is applied to the tip of the ski (Fig. 5.15) in a direction perpendicular to the ski, a moment will be produced at the ski binding. This moment tends to externally rotate the tibia. *Such a moment is called a torsional moment or torque.* We may think of torsional moments as moments that tend to produce internal or external rotation of the long bones.

### Moment Distribution

For the tibia under the loading condition imposed in Figure 5.15, equilibrium requires that the moment applied to the tibia at the knee joint be equal in magnitude but opposite in direction to the moment applied at the ski binding. If we choose to examine a distal segment of the tibia (Fig. 5.16), a free-body analysis shows that, for equilibrium, the moment applied to the internal cross-section of the tibia at the proximal end of the distal fragment must also be equal (in magnitude) to the applied moment but in the opposite direction. This internal torsional moment (torque) is applied by the distal face of the proximal fragment.

Using a convention analogous to that used in bending, we call these moments the internal torque. Note that the internal torque is constant throughout the length of the tibia. No matter what section of bone we choose to examine,

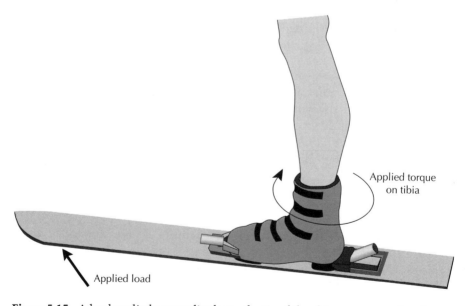

**Figure 5.15.** A load applied perpendicular to the tip of the ski creates a torsional moment (torque) that tends to externally rotate the tibia.

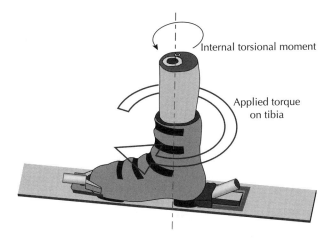

**Figure 5.16.** A free body of the distal tibia shows that equilibrium is satisfied if an internal torque of equal magnitude but opposite direction is applied at the upper boundary of the free body.

equilibrium conditions require the same internal torque to be present. This is in direct contrast to the bending moments produced by transverse loads. These internal bending moments are generally not constant, except in very special circumstances such as in the center sections of beams with symmetric four-point loading (Fig. 5.2). In torsional loading of the long bones, the internal torque is almost always constant along the length of the bone.

### Stress Distribution

What is the nature of the stresses acting on the internal surfaces of the tibia that produce the internal torque? To answer this question, let's examine a bar with a circular cross-section subjected to torsional loading (Fig. 5.17). The stress distribution on the internal circular cross-section, $A$, consists of a set of shear stresses that are greatest in magnitude at the periphery of the section and that diminish linearly toward the center of the section, at which point they are zero. If we term the shear stress at the outermost edge of the cross-section $\tau_{max}$, then in a manner analogous to the example used to describe bending, the shear stress at any point $r$ in the cross-section will be

$$\tau = \tau_{max} \times \frac{r}{R} \tag{5.11}$$

where $R$ is the outer radius.

The force caused by the shear stress acting on the small area $\Delta a$ will be equal to

$$F = \tau \times \Delta a$$

Again following our bending example, the amount of internal torque ($T_{Internal}$) produced by the force acting on area $\Delta a$ will be the force multiplied by the moment arm:

$$T_{Internal} = F \times r$$

To find the total internal torque, we sum the torques produced by all increments of area. This leads to the expression

$$T_{Internal} = \sum (\tau \times \Delta a) \times r$$

Substituting the proportionality for the stress (Equation 5.11), this expression becomes

$$T_{Internal} = \sum \left( \tau_{max} \times \frac{r}{R} \times \Delta a \right) \times r$$
$$= \frac{\tau_{max}}{R} \times \sum (\Delta a \times r^2) \tag{5.12}$$

The term $(\Delta a \times r^2)$ has special meaning. *The property of a circular cross-section derived from adding together the increments of cross-sectional area, $\Delta a$, each multiplied by the square of its distance from the center, $r^2$, is known*

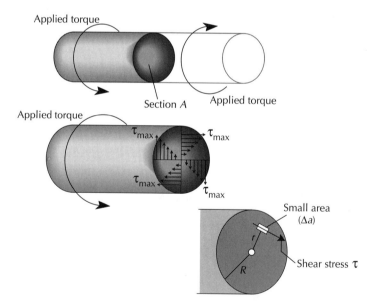

**Figure 5.17.** A circular bar of radius $R$ is loaded with a torsional moment. The shear stress distribution on section $A$ shows the magnitude of the stress at any point to be proportional to the distance to the point from the center of the bar. The shear stresses generate an internal torque equal in magnitude, but opposite in direction, to the applied external torque.

as the polar moment of inertia, $J$. This property of the cross-section is similar to the area moment of inertia, $I$ (Equation 5.5), but whereas $I$ is concerned with the distribution of area about a central axis (a line), $J$ is concerned with the distribution of area about a central point.

## Torsional Strength

If we wish to determine the maximum amount of torque ($T_{Ultimate}$) that can be applied to a structure without causing the structure to fail, we can use Equation 5.12. When the stress in the material reaches its failure value ($T_{Ultimate}$), we note that

$$T_{Ultimate} = \frac{\tau_{Ultimate} \times J}{R}$$

Note that the quantity $J/R$ is analogous to the section modulus, $I/(h/2)$, for the case of bending. This quantity is the proportionality constant between the maximum amount of torque that the structure can withstand, and the maximum shear stress ($\tau_{Ultimate}$). Recognize that, just as with bending strength, torsional strength depends upon a material property and a cross-sectional property. The material property is the ultimate shear stress that the material can tolerate, and the cross-sectional property is the torsional "section modulus," $J/R$. For a solid circular cross-section,

$$\frac{J}{R} = \frac{\pi \times R^3}{2}$$

Thus, the torsional strength will vary as the cube of the cross-sectional radius, $R$, a finding again similar to the bending strength for sections of this shape.

When we examined bending, we found that the concept of bending section modulus conveniently applied to all cross-sectional shapes. Unfortunately, this is not true for torsional loading. For sections that are not circular, the torsional "section modulus" cannot be easily computed. The reason for this lies in the nonlinear distribution of the shear stresses for noncircular cross-sections. This contrasts with bending, where stress distributions are linear regardless of the cross-sectional shape. For noncircular sections, the maximum shear stress, $\tau_{max}$, is usually not located at the portion of the cross-section that is farthest from the central point.

To illustrate nonlinear shear stress distribution, consider a bar with a square cross-section (Fig. 5.18). When the bar is subjected to torsional loading, the shear stress distribution shows the largest stresses to be at the centers of the faces of the square. The surfaces at the corners of the square carry no shear stress. Contrast the square cross-section with an almost circular cross-section (Fig. 5.19). This section differs from a circle only in that it has reentrant corners. Unlike the case for the corners of the square, the stress on the surface of the cross-section near the reentrant corners is very high. In general, outside corners such as fins and flutes carry little shear stress and hence contribute little to torsional strength. However, they are not detrimental. Reentrant corners, on the other hand, intensify the shear stress in the region of their most central projection and diminish the shear stress in the nearby outer regions of the sections. Thus, reentrant corners diminish the torsional load-carrying capacity of sections, acting somewhat like stress concentrations.

The effect of torsional loading on bars with a third type of geometry, usually termed an "open section," must also be understood. These sections defy intuitive analysis. To understand their torsional behavior, let's return to our previous example of a hollow circular intramedullary rod with an outside diameter of 14 millimeters and an inside diameter of 10 millimeters (see page 152). $J/R$, a measure of the torsional strength for this cross-section, can be calculated as

$$\left(\frac{J}{R}\right)_{\text{Hollow rod}} = \left(\frac{J}{R}\right)_{\text{14 mm rod}} - \left(\frac{J}{R}\right)_{\text{10 mm rod}}$$

$$= \frac{\pi \times (7 \text{ mm})^3}{2} - \frac{\pi \times (5 \text{ mm})^3}{2}$$

$$= 539 \text{ mm}^3 - 196 \text{ mm}^3$$

$$= 343 \text{ mm}^3$$

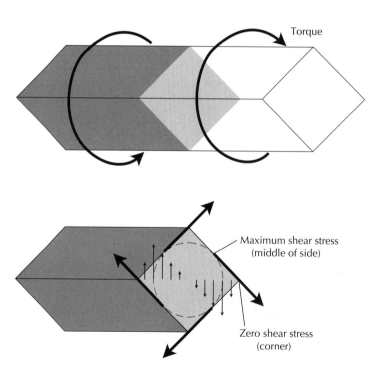

**Figure 5.18.** A bar with a square cross-section is subjected to torsional loading. The maximum shear stress does not occur at the corners, even though the corners are at the maximum distance from the center of the bar. Thus, the stress is not distributed linearly from the center of the bar.

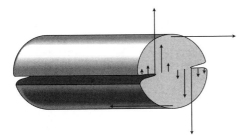

**Figure 5.19.** Reentrant corners in a cross-section cause the shear stress on the surface near the corner to be quite large compared with the stress if no corner were present in the cross-section. Note the non-linear distribution of shear stress.

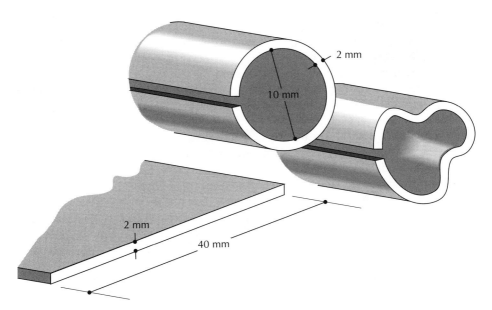

**Figure 5.20.** A flat plate bent into the shape of either rod shown will continue to exhibit the torsional strength of the flat plate as long as the open section remains. If the ends of the open section were welded together, the torsional strength (and stiffness) would be considerably greater.

If this same rod were manufactured by taking a flat plate 40 millimeters wide by 2 millimeters thick and of appropriate length, and bending it almost into a circle (Fig. 5.20), would the torsional strength of this rod be the same as the rod of the previous example? The answer, surprisingly, is no. The torsional strength of the fabricated tube will be the same as for the flat plate, unless the edges of the bent tube are welded together. In fact, no matter what shape the plate is bent into (for example, the cloverleaf in Fig. 5.20), the torsional strength of the section remains unaltered. The proportionality between the maximum torque, $T_{\text{Ultimate}}$, and the maximum shear stress, $\tau_{\text{Ultimate}}$, for the flat plate (analogous to $J/R$ for the circular cross-section) is

$$\frac{T_{\text{Ultimate}}}{\tau_{\text{Ultimate}}} = \frac{\text{Base} \times \text{Height}^2}{3}$$

$$= \frac{40 \text{ mm} \times (2 \text{ mm})^2}{3}$$

$$= 53 \text{ mm}^3$$

This value applies to the flat plate, the incomplete ring, and the cloverleaf. This measurement of strength is only about one-sixth that of the 14-millimeter-diameter hollow intramedullary rod.

A more intuitive sense might be gained by examining the stress distribution for the three configurations shown in Figure 5.21. For the continuous hollow cylinder, the shear stress distribution is similar to that of the solid cylinder in Figure 5.17. Note that the vectors representing each intensity level of stress form a closed loop, and each area of the surface has a force that produces a counterclockwise moment arm equal to the radius. For the flat plate, the shear stresses have a similar symmetric distribution. In this case, the moment arm for the forces produced by the stresses is, by comparison, quite small. Thus, a relatively small applied torque can produce relatively large-intensity stresses. When the plate is bent into the open-section cylindrical shape, the shear stress distribution does not change appreciably. While it may seem that the stresses at the outer surface now enjoy a larger moment arm with respect to the center of the cylinder, the shear stresses near the inner surface detract from this moment by producing a moment in the opposite direction. In fact, the difference in moments produced by the stresses located in the outer and inner regions, respectively, is virtually identical to the moment produced by the stresses in the flat plate.

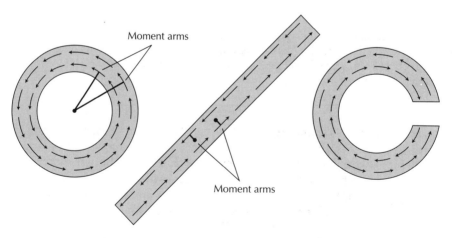

**Figure 5.21.** The stress distributions for a hollow rod differ from those of a flat plate and an open section.

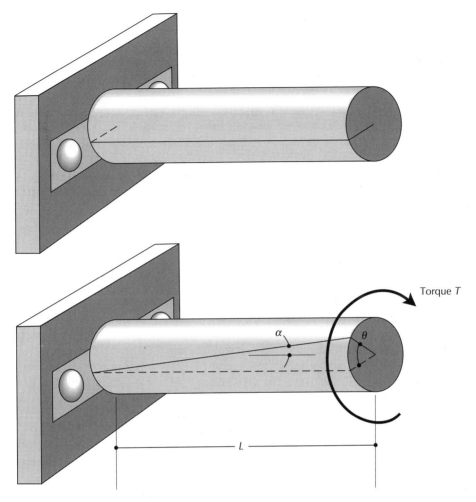

**Figure 5.22.** A circular cylinder is loaded about one end and has a torque applied to the other end. The torque causes an angle of twist $(\theta)$ to the rod.

## Torsional Rigidity

When torsionally unstable fractures of the long bones are treated with open reduction and internal fixation, the fixation device must transmit torsional as well as bending loads in a manner that allows fracture healing. Like bending loads, torsional loads can induce relative motion at the fracture site. Fixation devices must therefore be of sufficient torsional rigidity to prevent excessive fracture site rotation. To illustrate which properties of the structure control torsional rigidity, let's define terminology by considering the example shown in Figure 5.22.

We have applied torsional load to a circular cylinder and have noted the original and final configurations of three lines drawn on its surface. We consider one end of the cylinder to be fixed, and we note that the other end has rotated through an angle $\theta$ with respect to the fixed end. We further note that the line that was originally straight on the surface of the cylinder is now twisted into a helix. As we apply the external torsional load, the helix angle, $\alpha$, increases proportionally with the torque. We further observe that the helix is uniform over the entire length of the rod. The uniform helix angle indicates an equal contribution to total angular deformation from each increment of rod length. The total angular deformation, $\theta$, is also seen to be proportional to both the intensity of the applied torque and the length of the rod. We can observe this by substituting rods of different lengths but identical cross-section and repeating the experiment. We can therefore conclude that the angle of twist is proportional to the applied torque multiplied by the length of the rod:

$$\theta \propto T \times L$$

When discussing the behavior of beams, we found it convenient to define bending rigidity (see page 155). *We define torsional rigidity as the amount of torque required to produce a unit angle (one radian) of torsional deformation.* As with beams in bending, the proportionality constant between the torque and the angle of deformation depends upon two factors: a property of the material and a property of the structure's cross-section. The material property that controls the proportionality between torque and angle of twist is the shear modulus ($G$). The shear modulus for 316L stainless steel is 69 gigapascals, and that of cortical bone tissue is 3.3 gigapascals (Chapter 4, page 111). If two cylinders, one made of bone and one made of steel, have the same size and shape, the cylinder made of bone will have 21 times the torsional deformation of the one made from steel. Thus, the steel cylinder will be 21 times more rigid than the bone cylinder.

The structural property controlling the torsional rigidity is the polar moment of inertia ($J$) if the structure is a circular cylinder. If the shape is not a circular cylinder, the proportionality constant is not strictly $J$, but something related to it. The way of calculating this property depends upon whether the cross-sectional shape has external or reentrant corners and whether it is of open or closed section. For sections with outside corners (Fig. 5.18), the material in the corners adds little to the torsional rigidity. For open sections (Fig. 5.20), the torsional rigidity is virtually the same as for a flat plate of similar thickness and cross-sectional area.

Even though the proportionality constant between torque and angular deformation cannot be universally categorized for all cross-sections, there are nevertheless general rules that apply. The polar moment of inertia for a circular cross-section can be calculated as follows:

$$J = \frac{\pi \times R^4}{2}$$

We note that this property includes a shape dimension (radius) raised to the fourth power. If we were to evaluate the polar moment of inertia for a flat plate, we would find

$$I_{Plate} \propto \frac{Base \times Height^3}{6}$$

Note that this expression also contains a combination of characteristic dimensions raised to the fourth power. The same is true for any similar shapes (for example, squares). Thus, if we want to compare the torsional rigidities of similar shapes, we determine the characteristic dimensions, perhaps by looking in reference books (7), and compare ratios of the fourth powers of those dimensions. In general, just as in bending, if we double the cross-sectional size of the structure loaded in torsion, we will increase the rigidity by a factor of $2^4$. Contrast this with the increase in torsional strength, which would be $2^3$.

## Torque-Deflection Behavior

The torsional loading characteristics of a structure can be obtained from a curve of applied torque plotted against angular deformation, using much the same analysis as for beams in bending. If we examine the torque–versus–angular deformation curve of a tibia, we will usually observe an approximate straight-line region at the point of initial loading. The slope of the straight-line region ($\Delta$Torque/$\Delta$Angle) is the torsional rigidity of the structure. As for bending, we can also identify the fracture strength of the bone, as well as the maximum angular deformation to the point of failure.

Let's note in particular the area under the curve, which is proportional to the maximum torque multiplied by the maximum angular deformation. This quantity represents the amount of energy put into the bone by the externally applied torsional moment as the bone moves through the deformation angle. For the tibia, this area is 11 joules. Returning to Figure 5.15, we note that the skier has both kinetic energy (because of his velocity) and potential energy (because of the height of his center of gravity above the ground). We can calculate his kinetic energy from Equation 2.3, knowing his mass to be 80 kilograms and his velocity to be 20 kilometers per hour (5.6 meters per second):

$$Kinetic\ energy = \tfrac{1}{2} \times 80\ kg\,(5.6\ m/sec)^2$$

$$= 1254\ J$$

We can find the skier's potential energy from Equation 2.2, knowing that his center of gravity is 1 meter off the ground:

$$Potential\ energy = 785\ N \times 1\ m$$

$$= 785\ J$$

Comparing the energy that the tibia can absorb to the point of fracture with the available kinetic and potential energy of the skier's body, we again see that bone cannot effectively absorb a significant portion of the energy present during common traumatic events.

## *References*

1. Noyes FR, Butler DL, Grood ES, Zernicke RF, Hefzy MS. Biomechanical analysis of human ligament grafts used in knee-ligament repairs and reconstructions. J Bone Joint Surg 1984;66A:344-352.

2. Rybicki EF, Simonen FA, Mills EJ, Hassler CR, Scoles P, Milne D, Weis EB. Mathematical and experimental studies on the mechanics of plated transverse fractures. J Biomech 1974;7:377-384.

3. Carter DR, Vasu R. Plate and bone stresses for single- and double-plated femoral fractures. J Biomech 1981;14:55-65.

4. Frankel VH. The femoral neck: An experimental study of function, fracture mechanism and internal fixation. Uppsala: Almquist and Wiksells, 1960:74.

5. American Society for Testing and Materials. Standard test method for static bending properties of metallic bone plates (F382-86). In: Annual book of ASTM standards, section 13. Easton, Maryland: ASTM, 1990:74-77.

6. American Society for Testing and Materials. Standard practice for static bend and torsion testing of intramedullary rods (F383-73). In: Annual book of ASTM standards, section 13. Easton, Maryland: ASTM, 1990:78-79.

7. Roark RJ, Young WC. Formulas for stress and strain. 5th ed. New York: McGraw-Hill, 1975:290-296.

# 6

## Mechanical Behavior of Bone

**MECHANICAL BEHAVIOR OF BONE TISSUE**
**MECHANICAL BEHAVIOR OF WHOLE BONES**

## MECHANICAL BEHAVIOR OF BONE TISSUE

Since the skeleton is the basic structure on which our locomotive system is based, the mechanical behavior of this system is one of the most fundamental aspects of orthopaedic surgery and related disciplines. As we presented in Chapter 5, the mechanical behavior of a structure depends on both the size and the shape of the structure, as well as the mechanical properties of the materials of which it is composed. Knowledge of the properties of bone tissue is essential to understanding the behavior of whole bones. In Chapter 4 we described the tensile behavior, including the elastic modulus (Table 4.1), and the yield strength and ultimate strength (Table 4.2) of bone tissue. We described the viscoelastic nature of bone tissue (page 120) and showed that altering the rate at which load is applied affects its mechanical response. We also described the anisotropic nature of bone tissue (page 116) and showed that the mechanical properties depend upon the direction in which the tissue is loaded. We would now like to broaden our discussion of the mechanisms of bone tissue failure and healing.

### Effects of Density

Bone tissue appears in the skeleton in many microstructural forms. In infancy, cortical bone appears in both lamellar and haversian forms. In each of these forms, the tissue can have varying density. This density variation is almost always associated with a varying porosity of either a microscopic nature, as seen in the diaphysis of long bones, or a macroscopic nature, as seen in cancellous bone of the epiphyses. In general, the term *cortical bone* is used for bone tissue with a density greater than about 1.5 grams per cubic centimeter. Below about 1 gram per cubic centimeter, the bone is generally considered cancellous. Often the distinction is based on bone location rather than density, but this can lead to confusion, especially in those regions where very thin bony end plates exist.

If we examine the compressive behavior of bone tissue, we will find that the mechanical properties, as well as the failure mode, follow a continuum with respect to density. That is to say, a universal relation exists to express the compressive behavior of bone tissue as a function of density. For our first example, we will examine a piece of cortical bone removed from the mid-diaphysis of a human femur from an individual in the fourth decade of life. Its compressive behavior will generally be predictable and repeatable. The stress-versus-strain curve (Fig. 6.1) exhibits two regions. The first is an essentially linear, reversible, and, hence, elastic region; and the second is a nonlinear, irreversible, and, hence, plastic region. As described in Chapter 4 (page 124), multiple loading cycles within the elastic region can cause fatigue failure. But for single loading situations, the ultimate strength of the tissue is well represented by the peak load sustained by the piece of bone.

If a segment of cancellous bone, such as might be obtained from the tibial plateau, is similarly loaded in axial compression, a stress-versus-strain curve as shown in Figure 6.1 will result. As with our cortical bone specimen, if we load

**Figure 6.1.** A stress-versus-strain curve for human cortical bone tissue loaded in compression exhibits an initial linear, elastic region followed by a nonlinear, plastic region. A similar curve is obtained for cancellous bone tissue.

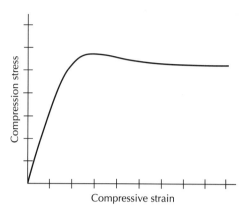

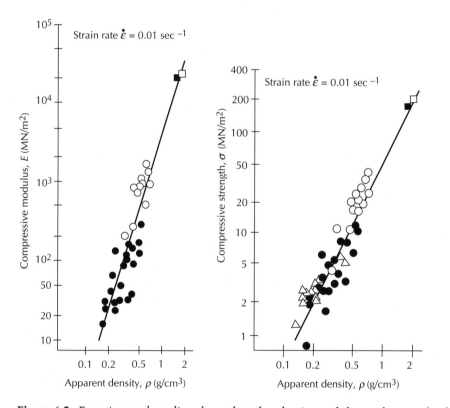

**Figure 6.2.** Experimental studies show that the elastic modulus and strength of bone tissue can be predicted from its density (1). Shown are human (filled) and bovine (open) bone tissue.

and unload the cancellous bone specimen within the initial straight-line region, elastic behavior is observed. For cancellous bone, the elastic modulus and the ultimate stress have been shown to correlate with the density ($\rho$, with typical units of grams/cubic centimeter) of the cancellous bone in the specimen (1). In fact, for bone tissue in general, the elastic modulus ($E$) correlates well with the cube of the density, and the ultimate stress ($\sigma_{ult}$) correlates well with the square of the density (Fig. 6.2):

$$E \propto \rho^3$$

$$\sigma_{ult} \propto \rho^2$$

Similar correlations have been observed between the elastic modulus and the degree of mineralization (the amount of mineral per unit weight), and between these properties and the total mineral content (the amount of mineral per unit volume) of the bone tissue (2).

### Effects of Age

Changes in the mechanical properties of bone tissue are noted to correlate with the age of the donor (3). Bone tissue from immature animals, as well as immature people, displays a lower elastic modulus, a lower tensile strength, and a higher total elongation to failure than tissue from more mature bone (Fig. 6.3). For human bone, as the age of the donor increases, both the elastic modulus and the yield strength increase up to about the third decade of life. Elongation to failure, however, decreases throughout life. In comparing average load-versus-deformation curves for mid-diaphyseal femoral bones from donors of different ages, we note that most mechanical properties decrease with age (Fig. 6.4). Associated with the decrease in mechanical properties is an increase in

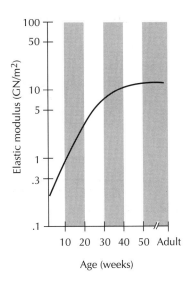

**Figure 6.3.** The modulus of elasticity of dog bone changes markedly with maturation. Similar changes occur in human bone (4).

**Figure 6.4.** Bone sampled from the midshaft of the femur shows properties that are age-dependent. The elastic modulus and yield strength decrease with age (3).

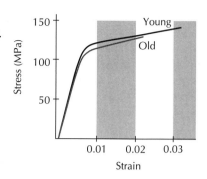

**Table 6.1.** Location Effects (3) of Cortical Bone Tensile Mechanical Properties (sixth decade of life)

|  | Yield Stress (MPa) | Ultimate Stress (MPa) | Elastic Modulus (GPa) |
|---|---|---|---|
| Femur | 111 ± 12 | 129 ± 6 | 17 ± 2 |
| Tibia | 124 ± 8 | 147 ± 9 | 20 ± 2 |

the porosity of bone tissue, a process that is positively correlated with aging. One property that remains rather constant with age is the elongation at which the bone achieves its yield strength.

## Effects of Location

Perhaps somewhat surprisingly, bone tissue properties also depend upon the anatomical region from which the bone is collected. Specimens of approximately equal density collected from the femur of an individual donor will have significantly different mechanical properties compared with specimens obtained from the tibia of the same individual (Table 6.1). There is also a detectable variation in mechanical properties around the circumference of the tibia or the femur. Depending upon the nature of the question being asked, such variation may be meaningful in the construction of analytical models to examine the behavior of bone structures.

## Effects of Species

When musculoskeletal research involves the use of other species, it is necessary to appreciate the difference in mechanical properties of the bone tissue. These properties have been catalogued for several species (2), and we show some selected data in Table 6.2. Note that most species have mechanical properties that exceed those of human bone. The ultimate strength of cortical bone tissue has been shown to correlate positively with bone mineral content. This correlation is observed across species (2).

**Table 6.2.** Species Effects of Elastic Properties of
Cortical Bone Tissue (2)

| Species and Source | Elastic Modulus (GPa) |
|---|---|
| Human femur | 18 |
| Cow femur | 23 |
| Sheep femur | 22 |
| Tortoise femur | 10 |
| Penguin humerus | 22 |
| Deer antler | 7 |
| Whale bulla | 31 |

## Failure Mechanisms for Bone Tissue

The method of treatment of fractures often depends in part on the injury mechanism. We can usually discover how a bone fractured by examining the bone tissue to determine its failure mode. For simple overload failure, bone exhibits distinct characteristics in tension, compression, and shear.

Tensile failure in bone tissue produces a crack perpendicular to the loading direction. The region of the crack is generally featureless, but the crack location within the microstructure depends upon the load orientation with respect to the orientation of the osteons. When load is applied in the longitudinal direction, the fracture surfaces are transverse to the osteons. Loads applied in the transverse direction produce fracture surfaces that can circumscribe the osteons for slow loading rates (Fig. 6.5) and transect the osteons for rapid loading rates.

As we observed from a tensile test of a bone specimen, bone tissue damage occurs when the yield stress has been exceeded but the rupture stress has not yet been reached. The nature of the damage to the tissue in the postyield (plastic) region is poorly understood. Yield is associated with the creation of microscopic porosity, a phenomenon that can be observed as a change in the bone's reflectivity and transmissibility of light. Thus, the creation of micropores is a phenomenon that has only been indirectly observed.

Compressive overload presents an entirely different type of failure mechanism. When bone tissue reaches the yield stress in compression, microscopic cracks form in and around the osteonal structure on planes that are approximately 45 degrees to the axis of loading. These cracks occur in increasing numbers as the load increases. When the load reaches a critical intensity, the small struts of bone separating the cracks collapse, giving the appearance of a larger, irregular crack. The gross orientation of this crack is also about 45 degrees to the loading axis. Continued loading increases the number of cracks, and eventually there is a slippage of the two fragments of bone adjacent to the biggest crack (Fig. 4.17). Recalling (from Chapter 4, page 106) that the maximum shear stresses are produced on surfaces that are oriented 45 degrees to the axis of tension or compression loading, we can attribute the formation of the microscopic cracks to the shear stresses. The surfaces that lie between the layers of the osteonal structure develop shear cracks in the presence of large shear stresses.

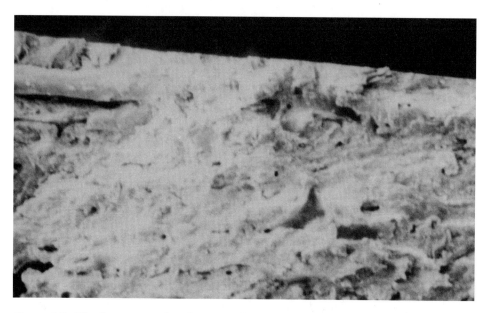

**Figure 6.5.** The fracture surface has completely isolated the osteon at the upper left corner of the tensile specimen.

**Figure 6.6.** Torsional loading of a bone specimen induces a longitudinal shear crack in the middle of the face of the square specimen. This crack then spirals around the specimen.

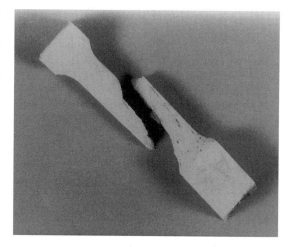

Thus, the mechanism by which bone fails under compressive loading is shear failure around and within osteons.

When bone is subjected to torsional loading, shear stresses are induced in the longitudinal and transverse planes. A compound failure mechanism occurs in which an initial crack is formed on a longitudinal surface. Since the specimen has a square cross-section, the maximum shear stress occurs at the center of the face (Fig. 5.18). This crack grows until it is about 1 or 2 millimeters long, it then changes direction to about 45 degrees to the longitudinal axis and spirals around the bone, and its ends are then joined by a much longer longitudinal crack (Fig. 6.6). While the initial crack is created on a plane of maximum shear stress, the continuing or spiraling crack is created on a plane of maximum tensile stress. The final closure of the spiral formed by the longitudinal crack is actually produced by bending, analogous to opening a book and cracking the binding.

## MECHANICAL BEHAVIOR OF WHOLE BONES

### Bending

When bending loads are applied to the long bone of a limb, the intensity of the compressive and tensile stresses induced are approximately equal. This is due to the relative symmetry of the bone. Because the yield and rupture stresses of bone tissue under tensile loading are much less than the yield and rupture stresses under compressive loading, the symmetry at the cross-section results in a failure that initiates in the region of highest tensile stress.

When the bone tissue reaches its tensile yield stress, it can continue to support additional induced stresses. If the bending load is increased, the tissue will respond with a slightly increased stress, albeit at a greatly increased strain. This has the effect of forcing the bone tissue in the rest of the cross-section to increase its stress more severely, in response to each increment of increasing bending moment (5). The bone therefore exhibits a nonlinear load-versus-deformation region, in which the slope of the curve (the bending rigidity) gradually decreases (Fig. 6.7).

Rupture of bone tissue under tensile stress does not occur until the tissue has elongated sufficiently to reach its ultimate stress. The general proportions of the load-versus-deformation curve for the bone indicate that the straight-line region (elastic behavior) extends to about half of the failure load of the whole bone. Thus, the bone continues to carry increasing bending load after the bone tissue begins to yield. Whereas the load can approximately double from the point of yield initiation to the rupture point, the area under the load-versus-deformation curve (which represents the absorbed energy) can more than triple.

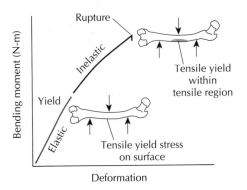

**Figure 6.7.** The curve showing load (bending moment) versus deformation for a whole femur loaded in bending is nonlinear. The bending rigidity (the slope of the curve) decreases as the deformation increases beyond the yield point.

Therefore, not all skeletal trauma falls into the two classifications of fully reversible bone loading and bone fracture. Some trauma results in permanent change in the shape of the bone (Fig. 6.8).

Since bone tissue's ability to yield is an important phenomenon in controlling bone strength, the loss of ductility that accompanies aging may be expected to have severe consequences. Fortunately, there are coincident changes in bone geometry that somewhat mitigate this effect. As an individual ages, bone tissue is resorbed from the endosteal surface of the cortex and bone tissue is laid down on the periosteal surface. Thus, the aging process is associated with thinner bones of larger diameter. The increase in diameter contributes to the bending strength as the cube of the diameter (or radius as in Chapter 5, page 152). This strengthening effect due to the change in the distribution of bone in the cross-section partly compensates for the weakening effect of the bone's decreasing ductility.

When the bending moment imposed on the bone causes the tissue opposite the loading point to exceed its rupture strength, a transverse crack is initiated (Fig. 6.9). The crack grows longer and starts to circumscribe the bone. Depending upon how rapidly the bending load is applied, the crack may remain a single crack or may bifurcate. The more rapidly the load is applied, the more the crack will bifurcate and the greater will be the number of resulting bone fragments. In fact, one of the methods by which the bone dissipates the large amount of

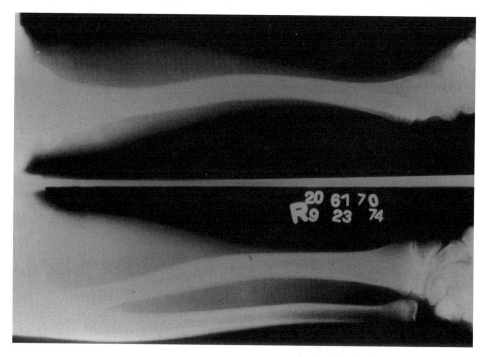

**Figure 6.8.** The bowed forearm resulted from the subject being on the bottom of a pileup during an informal football game.

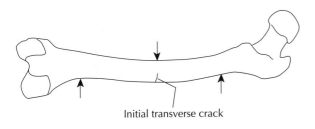

Initial transverse crack

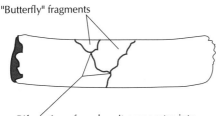

"Butterfly" fragments

Bifurcation of crack as it propagates into
the compression region of the bone

**Figure 6.9.** One of the ways a bone can dissipate energy applied during trauma is to fracture, thus creating free surfaces. The more energy there is to be dissipated, the larger the number of cracks generated within the bone.

energy being supplied to it under rapid loading is to create additional free bone surfaces through the creation of a large number of cracks. The number of fragments (the degree of comminution) is therefore directly related to the velocity of the impact.

In appearance, a bending failure always begins as a single transverse crack on the tensile side of the bone. For low-velocity injuries, the crack usually propagates across one-third to one-half the circumference of the bone, and it then becomes oblique at an unpredictable angle to the axis. At higher loading velocities, the bifurcation of the crack fragments (often called "butterfly" fragments) are produced in the central or lowest-stressed region of the bone's cross-section.

## Torsion

For a bone fractured in bending, the location of the bending load is always identifiable by its proximity to the site of fracture initiation. No such relationship exists between the point of application of torsional load and the torsional fracture site. Unlike bending, where the moments vary along the length of the bone, torsional loading produces a constant moment (Chapter 5, page 160). Therefore, fracture will form at whichever section produces the highest stress in response to the applied torque. We would axiomatically describe this location as the "weakest" section.

The location of the section in which torsional failure will be initiated can be determined by sampling a sufficient number of cross-sections and calculating which section has the lowest value of torsional "section modulus" (Chapter 5, page 163). The examination of the cross-sections' geometry allows the determination not only of the weakest section, but also of the actual location on the weakest section where the shear fracture will begin. Torsional fractures initiate at the outer surface that is closest to the centroid (the center of gravity) of the section (Figs. 5.18 and 6.6).

Tibial torsional fractures usually occur in the same location and have a characteristic appearance. This is because the tibia's weakest section usually lies near the junction of the middle and distal thirds. Examining the cross-sectional shape, we see it is triangular with broad, flat surfaces (Fig. 6.10). The portion of the circumference that is located closest to the centroid is labeled *A*. This is the initiation point of the shear crack in torsional loading.

This initial longitudinal shear crack is usually only 1 or 2 millimeters in length, but it may be 10 or more millimeters in length. The two secondary tensile cracks that originate from the shear crack start within a distance of 1 to 2 millimeters. Thus, even if the initial shear crack is longer, the spiraling tensile

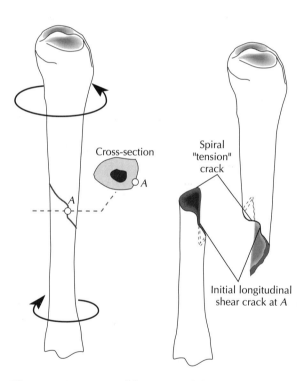

**Figure 6.10.** Torsional fractures of the tibia are initiated at the junction of the middle and distal thirds, where the strength of the cross-section is low because of its small dimensions. The initial shear crack propagates as two tensile cracks spiraling around the bone along directions perpendicular to the maximum tensile stress created by the applied external torque.

cracks expose only a small fraction of the shear surface (Fig. 6.10). The pattern of a spiral torsional fracture is also sensitive to how rapidly the torsional load is applied. Just as in bending, loads applied more rapidly produce more comminution. The comminution may appear as a double spiral, where more than two secondary tensile cracks originate from the initial shear crack. Another mode of comminution results from the bifurcation of one or more of the secondary tensile cracks.

## Effects of Altered Geometry

One of the most common biomechanical questions related to musculoskeletal rehabilitation concerns the weakening effect of surgically induced defects in the bone. Surgical intervention often leaves unfilled holes in bone. This is required, for example, by some compression plating techniques. Virtually all open reduction and internal fixation procedures with plates leave holes in the bone filled with screws. Similarly, the revision of a total joint prosthesis often requires the creation of a slot in the bone to remove acrylic bone cement. What happens to the strength of the whole bone in the presence of these defects?

Engineering theory states that the strain in the material adjacent to the hole will be two or more times higher than if the hole were not present. The increased strain in the bone tissue around a defect means that smaller torsional or bending loads are sufficient to initiate failure in these regions. The ratio of the failure load of the altered bone to the failure load of the intact bone is one measure of bone strength reduction.

In general, larger holes cause greater weakening. The amount of weakening produced by a hole depends not only on the size of the hole, but also on its location. For example, a hole near the proximal tibial plateau will not reduce the tibia's torsional strength. This is due to the large torsional "section modulus" of the proximal tibia as compared with the strength of the section at the distal-middle third junction. The shear strains induced in the larger, proximal section are less than one-third those induced in the distal section. Thus, the increased proximal section shear strain in the region of the hole does not exceed the strain induced simultaneously at the distal section. For a bending load applied at the midsection of a tibia, the strains created in the region of the hole in the proximal tibia are a small fraction of those in the region of the midshaft, where the fracture will occur. Thus, even doubling the strains in the proximal tibia will not induce failure at that site. Of course, if a failure is not induced at the hole site, then the hole site has not adversely affected the bone's strength.

Consider the less obvious situation in which a hole is located at the bending load site but oriented along the neutral axis. Again, the strains in the immediate vicinity of the hole are very small, and doubling these strains will not induce fracture at the hole. Thus, holes may occur in relatively stronger sections of bone, or in the low-stress regions of weaker sections, without appreciably affecting the bone's strength.

**Figure 6.11.** The torque-versus-angle curve for a torsion test of two bones, one with and one without a hole (6).

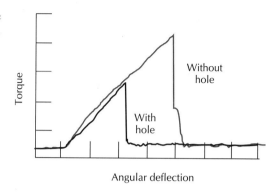

Whenever internal fixation produces holes in the region of the fracture site, the holes weaken the bone in loading situations that are similar to the original trauma. The original trauma identified the weakest section, which now, due to the surgical intervention, contains the holes. Experimental models have shown that, if the bone strength is measured using torsional loading immediately after surgery, screw holes reduce the torsional strength by slightly more than 50 percent (Fig. 6.11) (6). If the hole is left empty, the bones of experimental animals recover their full torsional strength in 8 to 12 weeks. If, at the time the hole is drilled in the bone, a screw is inserted (either self-tapping or pretapped), the time required for the bone to return to full strength is also 8 to 12 weeks. Removal of the screw after the bone has recovered its original torsional strength again results in a reduction in strength of about 50 percent. It seems that the screw damages the bone when it is removed, and this results in a weakening of the bone. Tests using bending loads to measure bone strength have shown that the hole weakens the bone only if it is located in the region of tensile stress opposite the bending load. Strength reduction is approximately 40 percent for a screw hole whose diameter is 30 percent of the bone diameter. Since the weakening effect of a hole is a function of its size, holes approaching 60 percent of the bone diameter cause a 55 percent strength reduction (7).

The process that allows the return of bone strength after the drilling of a hole, with or without insertion of a screw, appears to depend on remodeling and does not require the filling of the hole with bone tissue (6). The radiologic and morphologic appearances of the hole show that while remodeling and some filling of the hole occurs, the discontinuity is still present, even after the bone has regained its full strength. Remodeling of bone tissue around the hole is the most important aspect of the repair process, as was demonstrated in an animal experiment in which a drilled hole was filled with a polymeric plug. When the plug was removed at eight weeks, the torsional strength of the bone was normal even though the drilled hole was present.

The shape of the bone defect may influence the weakening effect. This influence is usually noticeable under torsional loading. If the defect is elongated in the direction of the bone axis, the weakening effect is greatly enhanced. For example, if the proximal tibia is used as a donor site for a bone graft (typically

20 percent of the length of the bone), torsional loads one-third or less of the load required to fracture an intact tibia cause torsional failure of the proximal tibia. If one considers that the strength in the proximal tibial cross-section is twice as great as a more distal cross-section near the junction of the middle and distal thirds of the tibia, the magnitude of the local strain at the graft defect can be appreciated. The local strain in the proximal tibia is increased at least sixfold. Such a defect of any shape, whether with rounded or square corners, severely reduces the strength of the bone in torsional loading (8). There may be small differences associated with rounded corners as compared with square corners, but these differences do not alleviate the gross weakening effect of the defect.

While we have used failure loads as a measure of bone strength, we have also shown that energy absorption can be indicative of bone strength (Chapter 5, page 159). Although the load-versus-deformation curves produced by both torsional and bending loads may not be linear, let's assume that they are for purposes of this discussion (see Fig. 6.11). We note that the reduction in torsional strength caused by a screw hole lowers both the load and the deformation to 50 percent of normal. Since the energy absorbed is represented by the area under the load-versus-deformation curve, and since the area for the triangular portion of the curve is one-half the product of the load multiplied by the deformation, the area (and hence the energy) is only

$$\text{Energy}_{\text{Defect}} = \frac{1}{2}[\text{Load}_{\text{Defect}} \times \text{Deformation}_{\text{Defect}}]$$

$$= \frac{1}{2}\left[\left(\frac{1}{2} \times \text{Load}_{\text{Intact}}\right) \times \left(\frac{1}{2} \times \text{Deformation}_{\text{Intact}}\right)\right]$$

$$= \frac{1}{4} \times \text{Energy}_{\text{Intact}}$$

For the case of the bone graft taken from the proximal tibia, reduction of the failure level of torque and angular deformation to one-third that for the intact tibia produces a similar result:

$$\text{Energy}_{\text{Graft}} = \frac{1}{2}[\text{Torque}_{\text{Graft}} \times \text{Angular deformation}_{\text{Graft}}]$$

$$= \frac{1}{2}\left[\left(\frac{1}{3} \times \text{Torque}_{\text{Intact}}\right) \times \left(\frac{1}{3} \times \text{Angular deformation}_{\text{Intact}}\right)\right]$$

$$= \frac{1}{9} \times \text{Energy}_{\text{Intact}}$$

In many situations, trauma can be quantified by the applied energy (Chapter 2, page 48). Therefore, if energy is considered as the strength criterion, the weakening effect of holes and slots is even more dramatic.

## Mechanical Aspects of Fracture Healing

The healing of fractured bone presents not only a biological challenge, but also a mechanical challenge. Healing must proceed in a manner that allows the earliest possible return to mechanical function, but without an excessive amount of reparative tissue. In the initial stages of normal bone healing, the bony fragments are bound by callus. While this material does possess some strength and stiffness, its elastic modulus is too low to make it useful in transmitting loads. Early stability in a healing fracture therefore requires compressive loads to be transmitted either through stabilized fracture fragments or through a mechanical fixation device.

During the early stages of healing, the bending and torsional strengths of an unfixed, stable fracture are low, typically 10 to 20 percent of the intact bone strength. The amount of gross deformation required to produce rupture of the callus is usually high, often greater than that for the intact bone. This is all the more remarkable since the major fragments of bone that constitute most of the bone's length have not appreciably decreased in stiffness. Yet in the presence of loads well below normal bone failure loads, the total deformation may easily exceed that of intact bone. This clearly indicates that the region of a fracture is many times less rigid than a normal section of bone. Thus, the earliest phase of fracture repair involves a mechanism that unites the fragments with a low elastic modulus and, hence, a low-rigidity envelope that has only moderate strength characteristics. The fracture site will still tolerate relatively large deformation without rupture of reparative tissues. Because deformation under load might be quite large, the energy required to produce failure in the early phases of healing is often comparable to that for intact bone.

In the next phase of the healing process, the callus undergoes calcification, whereby both its strength and its stiffness increase. The tissue can now support both tensile and compressive stresses, and the strength of the whole bone rapidly returns to its prefracture value. This restoration of strength occurs well before the callus tissue reaches the strength of normal bone tissue. The mechanism for restoration of strength is the production of a large volume of the weaker callus. The increased bulk of the tissue produces a large section modulus at the fracture site, and this allows restoration of bone strength. Although the strength of the bone may be near normal, the restoration of bone stiffness may lag. The low-elastic-modulus material of the callus produces sufficient deformation under load to keep the overall bone stiffness below normal. The amount of energy that the bone can absorb at this time may still exceed the energy absorption of the original intact bone.

The next phase of healing involves the final maturation of callus into a material whose strength and stiffness approximates that of normal bone. At this point, the bulkier callus produces a local section that is both stronger and stiffer compared with the prefracture condition. The whole bone will now appear grossly normal in response to mechanical loading. The final phase of healing involves remodeling and reformation of the bone at the fracture site. There are no mechanical consequences after this stage of the healing process.

### *References*

1. Carter DR, Hayes WC. The compressive behavior of bone as a two-phase porous structure. J Bone Joint Surg 1977;59A:954-962.

2. Currey J. The mechanical adaptations of bones. Princeton: Princeton University Press, 1984.

3. Burstein AH, Reilly DT, Martens M. Aging of bone tissue: Mechanical properties. J Bone Joint Surg 1976;58A:82-86.

4. Torzilli PA, Takebe K, Burstein AH, Zika JM, Heiple KG. The material properties of immature bone. J Biomech Eng 1982;104:12-20.

5. Burstein AH, Currey JD, Frankel VH, Reilly DT. The ultimate properties of bone tissue: The effects of yielding. J Biomech 1972;5:35-44.

6. Burstein AH, Currey JD, Frankel VH, Heiple KG, Lunseth P, Vessely JC. Bone strength: The effect of screw holes. J Bone Joint Surg 1972;54A:1143-1156.

7. McBroom RJ, Cheal EJ, Hayes WC. Strength reductions from metastatic cortical defects in long bones. J Orthop Res 1988;6:369-378.

8. Clark CR, Morgan C, Sonstegard DA, Matthews LS. The effect of biopsy-hole shape and size on bone strength. J Bone Joint Surg 1977;59A:213-217.

# 7

## Performance of Implant Systems

**LOAD SHARING**

**LOAD TRANSFER**

**CONTACT PROBLEMS IN TOTAL JOINT REPLACEMENT**

As in most medical disciplines, the growth in delivery of orthopaedic care has been strongly coupled with technological development. The major areas of technological growth in orthopaedic medicine have been in managing deformities, fractures, osteotomies, and the replacement of joint structures. Modern treatment of spinal deformities, for example, is strongly dependent on the use of implants. A large percentage of fractures are treated with open reduction and internal fixation. External fixation devices contribute to the management of complex fractures, as well as to postosteotomy treatment protocols such as leg lengthening. Hemijoint replacement and total joint replacement are excellent procedures for restoring joint function.

All of these devices share one functional feature. They must all transmit loads between biological structures. Some devices (such as compression plates or intramedullary rods) must transmit these loads while allowing a minimal amount of relative motion between the structures. Other devices (such as dynamic compression plates or external fixators for leg lengthening) permit a small but controlled amount of relative motion. Still other devices (such as hemijoint and total joint prostheses) are intended to allow large but confined motions. In order to provide a mechanism for load transfer, each of these devices must interface with the skeletal system at two locations. The interfaces are either with cortical bone, such as for a bone plate on the midshaft of the femur or the stem of the femoral component of a total hip replacement, or cancellous bone, such as in the femoral head for a sliding hip nail or in the proximal tibia for a total knee replacement. In each situation load transfer is accomplished either at discrete points, usually by screws or pins, or over broad surfaces, usually by press-fitting, cementing, or porous ingrowth. To have a stable interface with biological tissue, the implant structure must be designed so that the bone tissue at the interface is subjected neither to extremely high loads sufficient to cause local fracture or resorption nor to diminished loads that could induce local osteopenia.

The common mechanical feature of orthopaedic implant systems is their need to transfer load between the mechanical system and its biological interface. To understand and describe these systems, we recognize two distinct device types categorized by loading mechanism: load-sharing devices and load transfer devices. Load-sharing devices have structures that transfer load between the implant and the bone diaphysis. To understand this mechanism, consider the bone plate of Figure 5.1. This implant-bone interface is said to be load-sharing since at the portion of the plate at the fracture site all load is carried within the plate, and beyond the last attachment point (for example, the most distal screw) all load is carried by the bone. Between these two regions, some fraction of load is carried by the plate and the remainder is carried by the bone. The respective fractions carried by plate and bone will depend on the location between the fracture site and the last attachment point. Since the total load must be carried by both plate and bone, the load is said to be shared between the two structures. Other typical examples of load-sharing systems include well-fitted intramedullary rods and press-fitted or cemented stems of total hip replacement prostheses.

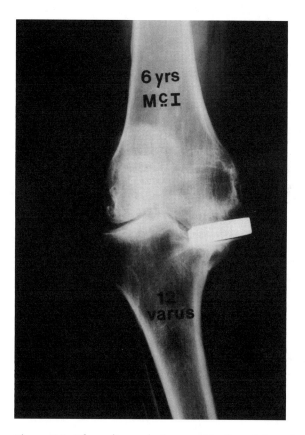

**Figure 7.1.** The radiograph shows a MacIntosh knee implant. It has a smooth, polished, slightly concave contact surface and is fabricated from cobalt alloy.

Load transfer devices transfer load between the implant and either the epiphysis of a long bone or the joint surface of a bone such as the pelvis or skull. Total load transfer occurs across the contact surface, but the distribution of contact pressure is often complex in geometry and depends upon the shape and rigidity of both the biological and mechanical structures. Some of the earliest implants that utilized load transfer surfaces were Smith-Petersen cups and MacIntosh tibial plateau inserts (Fig. 7.1). In both implants, the total joint contact load is transferred at each of the two interfaces—at the femoral and acetabular articulations for the cup, and at the femoral and tibial articulations for the plateau insert.

## LOAD SHARING

The concept of load sharing is important for understanding the performance of plates, rods, and stems. Control of load sharing is a vital design issue for the engineer, and predicting the biological consequences of load sharing is an integral part of patient management for the physician. The methods used to study load sharing in fracture fixation plates include direct measurement in animal models (1) and analytical techniques involving finite element models (2). While the details of performing analyses using finite element models are somewhat technical, the concepts are straightforward. Finite element modeling uses equilibrium concepts (Chapter 1) combined with a knowledge of the materials' stress-versus-strain behavior (Chapter 4). The same basic techniques that were used to find forces, moments, stresses, and strains for solid objects are applied to the finite element model. A free body is chosen that allows the investigation of all forces of interest. All forces crossing the free-body boundary must be considered. The process for determining the forces acting on the bone plate, as well as the displacements produced in the bone plate, is simplified by considering the plate to be an assemblage of small, bricklike elements. Depending upon the detail and precision required from the analysis, the brick elements may constitute a fine mesh (several thousand bricks in the model) or a coarse mesh (a dozen bricks in the model). No matter what the mesh size, each element obeys the rules of static equilibrium and is assigned appropriate elastic properties (elastic modulus, shear modulus, and Poisson's ratio), as well as appropriate failure properties (yield stress and ultimate stress).

The model's complexity depends upon the number of features the investigator wishes to include in the experiment. For example, if the bone plate model is to include the bone screws with sufficient detail to represent the threads, many elements must be utilized, and the complexity will grow. If the investigator wishes to include a fibrous tissue interface between the screws and the bone, additional elements possessing the elastic properties of fibrous tissue must be interposed between the screw thread and the bone. The model's complexity depends, therefore, upon the performance questions asked by the investigator and the properties or model variables that the investigator believes are important in controlling the model performance. If the investigator wishes to determine the motion of the screw threads relative to the bone, features of the thread geometry have to be incorporated into the model, increasing the complexity. Similarly, if the effect of the plate's surface roughness on the mechanical behavior of the bone-plate interface is to be examined, more complex interface elements that model the effect of friction must be used.

The loading that is applied to the structure must also be included in the model. External loads, such as joint contact forces, as well as internal forces that act across free-body boundaries are applied to the surfaces of the finite element model. Sometimes these forces are known, as would be the case for joint contact forces. In some situations the forces are unknown, as would be the case with internal forces. These forces must be determined as part of the solution.

Once we choose the model's geometry, including the shape and number of elements and their elastic and failure properties, and input the boundary conditions, including known and unknown forces, we can exercise the model using standard computational methods. Each computer-derived solution of a finite element model is analogous to the mean response of an experiment on a biological model. If the effects of additional variables, such as different elastic moduli, are to be studied, the finite element model can be modified to incorporate the variable changes, and additional solutions can be produced. This is analogous to changing variables in a biological model. Appreciation of both finite element models and biological models does not necessitate a detailed understanding of the internal processes involved in either model.

The finite element model that we wish to examine in understanding load sharing consists of an acrylic tube used to model the diaphyseal portion of an intact long bone, a bone plate, and cortical bone screws (3). This model allows us to conduct an experiment with a physical model in the laboratory and compare the solution of the finite element model with the laboratory results (Fig. 7.2). The choice of the acrylic tube allows a "standard," homogeneous structure to be examined, providing the closest possible match between the geometry and properties of the finite element model and the laboratory model. We will subject the model to a bending load of 9.3 newton-meters induced by two transverse loads and two supporting loads (Fig. 5.1).

If we first examine the stresses imposed on the tube in the absence of the bone plate, we see that with our simple, uniform-cross-section tubular model, we experience a symmetric stress distribution, with tensile stress on the superior surface equal to 8.5 megapascals and an equal-magnitude compressive stress on the inferior surface (Fig. 7.3).

If we now attach the bone plate to the tube's central region and again apply a unit bending load, we experience a dramatic change in the stress distribu-

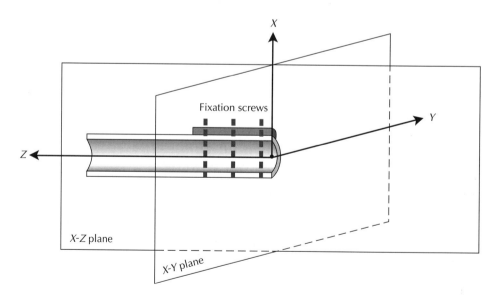

**Figure 7.2.** The tube in the model is used to represent bone. Half of the model is shown because of the symmetry of the problem.

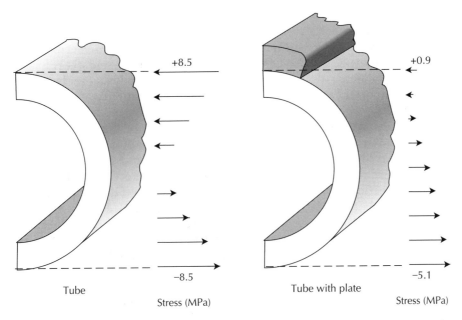

**Figure 7.3.** The cross-sections of the tube in both the unplated and plated conditions are shown. Compression stress is decreased in the bone opposite the plate, and tensile stresses are virtually eliminated in the bone under the plate (3).

tion. The "bone tissue" immediately under the plate experiences a maximum tensile stress only about one-tenth as large as in the unplated model. Most of the material in the tube is under compressive stress, with the neutral axis shifted from the tube's center to a point just below the bone plate. This is due to the equilibrium requirement that forces produced by the stresses on the cross-sectional area of both tube and bone plate must sum to zero. Thus, the compressive stresses in the tube's inferior region multiplied by the cross-sectional area below the neutral axis must be equal (but opposite in direction) to the tensile stresses in the tube's superior region and in the plate, multiplied by the respective tube and plate cross-sectional areas. Since the stresses in the plate will be greater than the stresses in the tube, more area of the tube must be subjected to compressive stress to allow the force balance required for equilibrium. Hence, the neutral axis moves from the center of the tube toward the plate, placing more of the tube under compressive stress.

Since the combination of the plate and the tube is stronger than the tube alone, the magnitude of the compressive stress in the tube decreases. Thus, the maximum stress in the tube model, located in the most inferior portion of the cross-section, has been reduced by 45 percent. We note that most of the cross-section of the tube model under the plate is now subject to compressive stress. This analysis is applicable to the situation in which a bone fracture has at least partially healed, since the cross-section under the plate is also carrying a small tensile stress. The maximum compressive stress in the tube has been reduced, as well as the maximum tensile stress. This indicates that the tube is no longer carrying all of the moment. The bending moment is being shared with the plate.

When we examine the experimental strain gauge results from the laboratory test on the acrylic tube, we find the same stress amplitude and distribution. This gives us confidence that the finite element model analysis can depict the effects of the important variables in a model containing a tubular structure and a bone plate. We would now be justified in applying this type of analysis to a model with the actual geometry and material properties of a bone.

The second example of a load-sharing device that we will examine is a press-fit intramedullary rod. We will start by considering only rods of uniform round cross-section. For a smooth polished rod, relative motion between rod and bone in the axial direction is not restricted. This means the rod does not transmit axial load to the bone. Smooth, round-cross-section intramedullary rods cannot transmit torsional loads to the bone, since shear stresses cannot be developed at the smooth interface between the rod and the endosteal bone surface. The only loads that the smooth cylindrical rod can transmit to the bone are the loads producing bending moments, since these loads are perpendicular to the smooth surface.

Thus, in the loading situation shown, the intramedullary rod shares bending moment in the proportion shown (Fig. 7.4). The rod models the behavior of either the stem of a total hip joint or an intramedullary fracture fixation rod. Note that much of the bending moment is carried by the rod throughout the

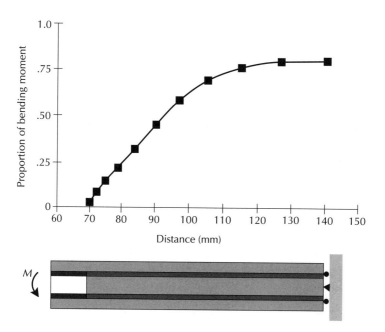

**Figure 7.4.** Distributions of bending moments acting on the stem at each cross-section for a cemented stem that is not bonded at the stem-cement interface.

rod's length. But as we near the tip of the rod, we see a more rapid transition, with a large fraction of the bending moment transmitted to the bone over a short distance.

To understand load distribution in these situations, it is necessary to appreciate the stiffness of each component of the system. In this case, we have a composite structure consisting of a rod and a bone subjected to bending. We realize that because of the intimate contact between bone and rod, bending of the composite structure produces the same deformation or curvature in the bone as in the rod. However, the bone and the rod have different bending stiffnesses. Therefore, to produce equal deformations, the bone and the rod require *unequal* bending moments. Specifically, for the more rigid rod, a higher bending moment is required to produce the same deformation compared with the less rigid bone. In fact, the magnitude of the bending moments in the rod or in the bone required to produce the same deformation in each component of the composite system is directly proportional to each component's bending stiffness. Thus, for load sharing in bending, each component captures that fraction of the total bending moment that represents its contribution to the total bending stiffness of the composite structure. If the bone has a stiffness of 1 newton-meter$^2$ and the rod has a stiffness of 2 newton-meters$^2$, the stiffness of the composite is the sum of the two, or 3 newton-meters$^2$. The bone has one-third of the composite stiffness, and the rod has two-thirds.

If we apply a 10-newton-meter bending moment, then one part in three of the moment ($3\frac{1}{3}$ newton-meters) is carried by the bone and two parts ($6\frac{2}{3}$ newton-meters) are carried by the rod. Thus, the moment carried by the bone is

$$\text{Moment}_{\text{Bone}} = \left(\frac{\text{Stiffness}_{\text{Bone}}}{\text{Stiffness}_{\text{Total}}}\right) \times \text{Moment}_{\text{Total}}$$

$$= \left(\frac{1\ \text{N} \cdot \text{m}^2}{3\ \text{N} \cdot \text{m}^2}\right) \times 10\ \text{N} \cdot \text{m}$$

$$= 3\,\tfrac{1}{3}\ \text{N} \cdot \text{m}$$

And the moment carried by the rod is

$$\text{Moment}_{\text{Rod}} = \left(\frac{\text{Stiffness}_{\text{Rod}}}{\text{Stiffness}_{\text{Total}}}\right) \times \text{Moment}_{\text{Total}}$$

$$= \left(\frac{2\ \text{N} \cdot \text{m}^2}{3\ \text{N} \cdot \text{m}^2}\right) \times 10\ \text{N} \cdot \text{m}$$

$$= 6\,\tfrac{2}{3}\ \text{N} \cdot \text{m}$$

Simply put, the stiffer component of the composite carries the greater share of the load.

The next increment of complexity that can be added to a load-sharing system is a mechanism to allow the transference of axial load. One mechanism by which an intramedullary rod can transmit axial load is the imposition of a layer of PMMA between the rod and the endosteal bone surface, as is done for cemented femoral stems in total hip replacement. If, in addition to the PMMA, the surface of the stem is either tapered or textured, axial load transfer can be enhanced. The mechanism of axial load distribution is similar to that for bending moments. If the intramedullary stem is well coupled to the bone surface, then the foreshortening caused by the compressive load will be the same in the intramedullary stem, the PMMA column, and the bone. This means that, as in load sharing with bending moments, the amount of axial load required to produce equal foreshortening in each unit length of each component will be proportional to that component's stiffness.

The axial stiffness of each component is equal to the component's cross-sectional area, multiplied by the elastic modulus of the material from which the component is made, divided by the length of the component (Equation 5.4). We have measured the area of the bone to be 905 square millimeters, the area of the PMMA to be 302 square millimeters, and the area of the 316L stainless steel intramedullary stem to be 314 square millimeters. While these areas are certainly not equal, they do not differ by the same magnitude as the elastic moduli of these three materials (see Table 4.1). The axial stiffnesses for each millimeter of length for the three components are

$$\text{Axial stiffness} = \frac{E \times A}{l}$$

$$\text{Axial stiffness}_{\text{Bone}} = \frac{(18 \text{ GPa}) \times (9.05 \times 10^{-4} \text{ m}^2)}{0.001 \text{ m}}$$

$$= 16.3 \times 10^9 \text{ N/m}$$

$$\text{Axial stiffness}_{\text{PMMA}} = \frac{(3 \text{ GPa}) \times (3.02 \times 10^{-4} \text{ m}^2)}{0.001 \text{ m}}$$

$$= 0.9 \times 10^9 \text{ N/m}$$

$$\text{Axial stiffness}_{\text{Stem}} = \frac{(180 \text{ GPa}) \times (3.14 \times 10^{-4} \text{ m}^2)}{0.001 \text{ m}}$$

$$= 56.5 \times 10^9 \text{ N/m}$$

The differences in elastic moduli are an overwhelming factor in controlling the differences in axial stiffness among the components within the composite structure. Note that the combined axial stiffness of all three components is only slightly greater than that of the intramedullary stem.

We may now determine the way in which axial load is shared by multiplying the total axial load by the percentage of total axial stiffness contributed by each component. Thus, for a 500-newton axial load, the load in the bone, PMMA, and stem will be

$$\text{Load}_{\text{Bone}} = \left(\frac{\text{Stiffness}_{\text{Bone}}}{\text{Stiffness}_{\text{Total}}}\right) \times 500 \text{ N}$$

$$= \frac{16.3 \times 10^9 \text{ N/m}}{73.7 \times 10^9 \text{ N/m}} \times 500 \text{ N}$$

$$= 111 \text{ N}$$

$$\text{Load}_{\text{PMMA}} = \left(\frac{\text{Stiffness}_{\text{PMMA}}}{\text{Stiffness}_{\text{Total}}}\right) \times 500 \text{ N}$$

$$= \frac{0.9 \times 10^9 \text{ N/m}}{73.7 \times 10^9 \text{ N/m}} \times 500 \text{ N}$$

$$= 6 \text{ N}$$

$$\text{Load}_{\text{Stem}} = \left(\frac{\text{Stiffness}_{\text{Bone}}}{\text{Stiffness}_{\text{Total}}}\right) \times 500 \text{ N}$$

$$= \frac{56.5 \times 10^9 \text{ N/m}}{73.7 \times 10^9 \text{ N/m}} \times 500 \text{ N}$$

$$= 383 \text{ N}$$

The load distribution at the stem tip is not predictable by this method of analysis. Figure 7.5 shows the result of a finite element model analysis of a stem-cement-bone system carrying axial load. The graph shows the load carried by each element of the composite system. Note that through most of the stem's

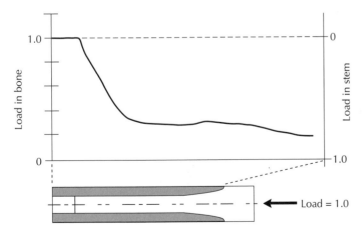

**Figure 7.5.** The pattern of load sharing is controlled by the relative stiffness of the components, except near the tip of the stem, where the pattern becomes irregular.

length, axial load is shared in proportion to the element's contribution to the total axial stiffness of the system. However, as we near the stem tip, the shared load displays an irregular pattern. Such findings are common at the transition points in composite structures.

Reconstructing the diaphyseal bone into a composite load-sharing system always results in a decrease of the load share carried through the bone. Both animal experiments and analysis have verified this phenomenon (1, 4). Since one of the fundamental biological laws is Wolff's law, there is considerable concern over the long-term implications of load sharing. The biological control mechanisms that produce the effects described by Wolff's law are as yet poorly understood. What is known is that in situations where bone loads are reduced or eliminated, bone mass is resorbed. If bone mass is resorbed in the load-sharing diaphyseal region, the bone stiffness will decrease. As can be appreciated from the previous analyses, decreasing the bone stiffness in the presence of an implant will result in less of the shared load being carried by the bone. This in turn will lead to further reduction in bone mass. Fortunately, the biological control system does not push most load-sharing bone implant systems to the extreme that this process would suggest. However, well-bonded intramedullary stems can often produce remarkable resorption by the mechanism of load sharing (Fig. 7.6).

We have seen how load sharing causes an appreciable fraction of the bending moment to be carried by an intramedullary stem. Now let's consider a possible failure mechanism for the stem of a well-fixed, cemented 316L stainless steel femoral component of a total hip replacement (5). Consider the peak loads during a gait cycle. The bending moment imposed by the combined effect of joint contact force at the acetabulum and the pull of the gluteus maximus muscle at the greater trochanter is 140 newton-meters at the cross-section where the fracture is located on the stem shown in Figure 7.7. This moment must be shared by bone, PMMA, and stem. The bending stiffness (elastic modulus multiplied by area moment of inertia) for each of these components is 293 newton-meters$^2$, 3 newton-meters$^2$, and 120 newton-meters$^2$, respectively, for a total composite bending stiffness of 416 newton-meters$^2$. The amount of moment that the stem will support is equal to

$$\text{Moment}_{\text{Stem}} = \frac{(E \times I)_{\text{Stem}}}{(E \times I)_{\text{Composite}}} \times 140 \ \text{N} \cdot \text{m}$$

$$= \frac{120 \ \text{N} \cdot \text{m}^2}{416 \ \text{N} \cdot \text{m}^2} \times 140 \ \text{N} \cdot \text{m}$$

$$= 40.3 \ \text{N} \cdot \text{m}$$

Recall that the maximum stress induced in a beam is equal to the applied bending moment divided by the section modulus (Equation 5.6). For the stem,

$$\text{Section modulus} = \frac{I}{c}$$

$$= 1.33 \times 10^{-7} \ \text{m}^3$$

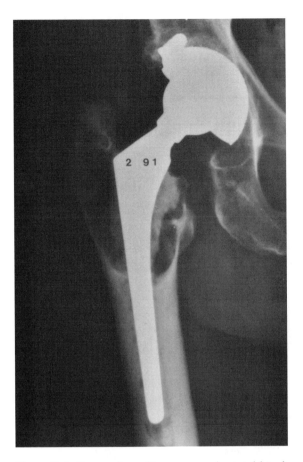

**Figure 7.6.** Resorption of bone around a total hip femoral component is evident on the radiograph. The bone resorption may be caused by a combination of load sharing and biological reaction to wear debris.

Therefore,

$$\text{Maximum stress} = \frac{\text{Moment}_{\text{Stem}}}{I/c}$$

$$= 303 \ \text{MPa}$$

When the maximum stress induced in the well-fixed stem is compared with the yield stress of the 316L stainless steel, we see that the induced stress represents an appreciable fraction of the yield stress. As shown in Table 4.3, the endurance limit of stainless steel is about half the yield stress (Table 4.2). Thus, the induced stress in the stem of a well-cemented prosthesis is near the stress magnitude required to produce fatigue failure.

Observe the continuity of the stem in Figure 7.7A. A slight irregularity can be seen along the lateral edge of the stem in the left femur. This patient

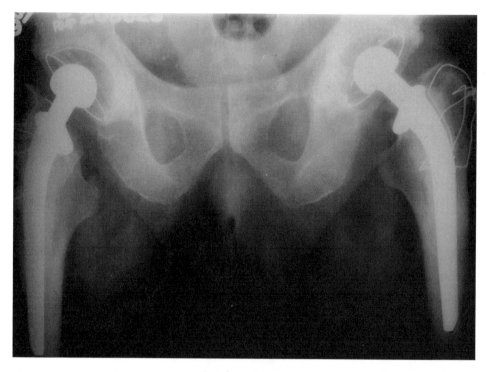

**Figure 7.7.** *A.* A radiograph of a patient with a fractured femoral prosthesis. *B.* The fractured cross-section was located at the junction of the proximal one-third and the distal two-thirds of the stem portion. The surface shows "clamshell" markings emanating from the anterolateral corner.

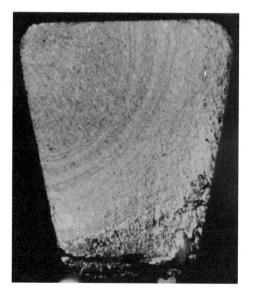

**Figure 7.7*B.***

complained of a sudden onset of localized thigh pain. At the time of surgery, the stem was found to have fractured, though both proximal and distal fragments were found to be well fixed. While fractured femoral stems are often associated with mechanical loosening, a stem does not have to be loose to experience sufficient cyclic stresses (through load sharing) to cause fatigue failure.

## LOAD TRANSFER

The introduction of surface replacements for hemi- and total joint prostheses created a new load transfer mechanism between prosthetic components and bone. These prostheses and their contemporary counterparts have broad areas of contact with the epiphyseal cancellous bone. Often they include supplemental fixation devices, such as stems, pegs, or screws. The mechanics of load transfer between these devices and the cancellous bone bed differ from that of load-sharing devices. Load transfer devices receive joint load in the midregion of the structure (Fig. 7.1). This load must be transferred across the device to the cancellous bone bed. In essence, the entire load imposed upon the device is carried within the device until the load transfers to the supporting cancellous bone.

In analyzing the mechanism of load transfer, our primary concerns center on three questions:

1. How is the load distributed on the implant by the contacting joint surface? Note that the contacting joint surface may be another implant structure, such as the femoral ball in a total hip replacement contacting the acetabular cup, or a natural joint surface, such as the distal femoral condyle contacting a MacIntosh tibial plateau insert.

2. How does this load distribution interact with the implant to change its shape? Remember that implants include thin metallic devices, such as the Smith-Petersen cup, and even more flexible tibial plateaus constructed from polyethylene. Loads imposed at joint surfaces, as well as those created at the prosthesis-bone interface, can readily distort these prostheses.

3. How do the combined effects of joint load and prosthesis distortion control the load distribution at the prosthesis-bone interface? Since the major requirement for any joint replacement implant is that it develop a stable prosthesis-bone interface, the manner in which load is transferred between prosthesis and bone is critical.

Load distribution and hence the contact stresses on the articular surface of load transfer implants depend upon the shape of the contacting surfaces and the elastic moduli of the contacting materials. For thin implants constructed of low-modulus materials or implants whose contacting surfaces have greatly differing elastic moduli, the thickness of the component also influences the load distribution at the contacting surface. To illustrate the effects of surface geometry, elastic modulus, and thickness on contact stresses, let's compare three

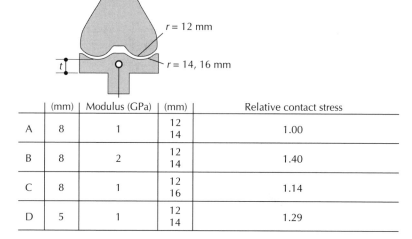

| | (mm) | Modulus (GPa) | (mm) | Relative contact stress |
|---|---|---|---|---|
| A | 8 | 1 | 12<br>14 | 1.00 |
| B | 8 | 2 | 12<br>14 | 1.40 |
| C | 8 | 1 | 12<br>16 | 1.14 |
| D | 5 | 1 | 12<br>14 | 1.29 |

**Figure 7.8.** The radius of curvature of the contacting surfaces, the modulus of elasticity of the polyethylene, and the thickness of the component all affect the contact stress in a total knee tibial component. The contact stresses for cases *B*, *C*, and *D* are compared to *A*.

systems (6). Our standard of comparison is the shape, elastic modulus (1 giga-pascal), and thickness (8 millimeters of polyethylene) corresponding to a conventional, modern condylar knee replacement (Fig. 7.8*A*). We have distributed the joint load equally between the two condyles. We contrast the resulting contact stress distribution with that produced by the same implant geometry, but with the elastic modulus of the polyethylene component doubled, as would be the case with an "enhanced" polyethylene material. In these circumstances, the peak contact stresses increase by 40 percent (Fig. 7.8*B*). For our next system, we retain the material properties of the example in part *A* but decrease the conformity of the polyethylene component. We have, in effect, made the tibial plateau component flatter. This change increases the peak contact stress by 14 percent (Fig. 7.8*C*). For our last illustration, we maintain the curvature and material properties of part *A* but decrease the polyethylene thickness from 8 millimeters to 5 millimeters. The peak contact stresses increase by 29 percent (Fig. 7.8*D*).

Since the contact stresses imposed on a prosthesis by joint loading are sensitive to the shape of the contacting surfaces, the actual contact geometry must be controlled for all conditions of joint function. As we saw in Chapter 3, not all possible positions of a stable knee joint produce a uniform sharing of joint load between medial and lateral compartments. For example, when the knee joint is loaded by both a flexion moment and a varus moment, the load may be totally concentrated on the medial plateau (Fig. 3.18). If extreme varus moments are applied, the lateral plateau may separate from the lateral femoral condyle, producing a lateral gap of 3 to 5 millimeters.

Let's examine the load distribution induced by 3 degrees of varus angular rotation of the tibial component. We will examine two surface geometries, one of constant radius (Fig. 7.9*A*) and one composed of 3 radii (Fig. 7.9*B*). Stress distributions for these two surface geometries are similar for the condition of equal loading on medial and lateral condyles. However, when the two prostheses are compared in the more severe loading state involving 3 degrees of varus angular rotation, the constant-radius geometry has a much less severe stress distribution. In fact, the stress distribution of the constant-radius geometry does not change with 3 degrees of varus angulation. The same cannot be said for the variable-radius geometry. Since the major inhibitor to the longevity of total knee prostheses is wear of polyethylene components, all possible design parameters that contribute to high surface stresses should be examined. In this case, we see that what appears to be a reasonable or even desirable surface geometry (that is, relatively flat surfaces) produces reasonable stresses under only one of many normally encountered conditions. Flat surface geometries

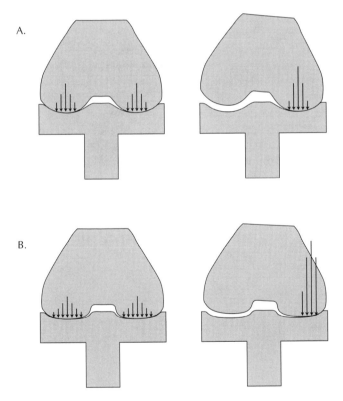

**Figure 7.9.** Two designs of total knee replacement are shown. *A*. In this design each plateau consists of a single medial-lateral radius of curvature. *B*. In this design each plateau consists of three radii of curvature in the medial-lateral direction (a large radius forming a nearly flat surface, with smaller radii of curvature at both edges). When the joint contact load is evenly distributed between both plateaus, design *B* shows a larger contact area (less severe load distribution) than design *A*. When sufficient varus or valgus moment is applied so that all the load shifts to one plateau (right), the load is much more concentrated for design *B*.

that are conforming under only one loading condition do not satisfy the need for controlling contact stresses under the many varied conditions encountered *in vivo*.

The distortion of the implant caused by the surface loads profoundly influences the load transfer pattern between the implant and the supporting cancellous bone bed. With most implant designs, the contacting surfaces between implant and cancellous bone are initially conforming. This applies to the flat undersides of tibial plateaus, as well as to the spherical outer surfaces of acetabular cups. If load transfer at these interfaces is to be uniform, the shape of the prosthesis should not change appreciably under load. To understand the interaction between surface loads, implant rigidity, and load transfer at the prosthesis-bone interface, we will examine a simple model of a tibial plateau. In this example we will consider all load applied on one condyle. In Figure 7.10*A* we depict a tibial plateau of 8 millimeters thickness, but with an exaggerated medial-lateral width. In Figure 7.10*B* we scale the medial-lateral width to an average anatomical size, and in Figure 7.10*C* we produce an abnormally narrow medial-lateral width.

When the load is applied to the joint surface of the plateau in Figure 7.10*A*, contact forces develop at the prosthesis–cancellous bone interface. The area over which these prosthesis-bone contact forces occur is broader than the area of the contact forces on the joint surface. This creates a bending moment distribution in the implant that tends to cause concave-upward deformation. The deformed prosthesis is no longer contiguous with the bony surface. Depending upon the attachment mode between the prosthesis and the bone, there may be no load transfer in the regions where separations occur, as, for example, in

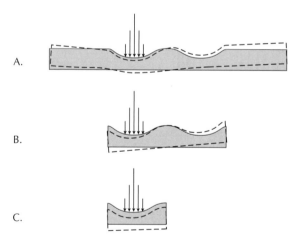

**Figure 7.10.** Three tibial plateaus with different medial-lateral widths are all supported by underlying cancellous bone and are all loaded by one condyle only. All three plateaus experience bending deformations, though the amount of deformation is greatest in the plateau with the largest medial-lateral dimension.

the case of cemented prostheses with no interlocking surfaces on the tibial plateau. Other attachment modes, such as cement interlocking, cement bonding, or porous surface bone ingrowth, may allow the development of tensile forces at this interface. In these cases, the load distribution at the prosthesis–cancellous bone interface will contain tensile forces, and the deformation pattern will be altered. Therefore, total joint components that are relatively thin can have complex load transfer patterns that depend upon the thickness-to-width ratio of the component, as well as upon the conditions of surface attachment.

If we examine the normal-size plateau (Fig. 7.10B), we see that the tendency to deform the plateau in a concave-upward direction still exists. However, because of the relatively shorter width, as compared with the thickness, only a small amount of separation occurs at the extreme lateral corner for the un-bonded case. For the bonded situation, tensile forces will be developed at the lateral edge with an associated decrease in the amount of lift-off.

Examining the reduced-width tibial plateau (Fig. 7.10C), which we can think of as representing a unicondylar component, we note that the bending effect is minimized because of the narrow plateau width (recall from Chapter 5 that the amount of bending deformation in a beam varies with the cube of its length). With its narrow medial-lateral width (that is, short beam length), the tibial plateau transfers load to the cancellous bone interface in an almost uniform manner. Unfortunately, whenever there is a region of sudden change in load distribution on a contact surface, high shear stresses are induced. Thus, under the lateral edge of the medial tibial plateau, we have a condition where the contact load abruptly changes intensity. This induces high shear stresses in the bone.

We can now define the ideal shape for a total joint surface replacement component. The length-to-thickness ratio should be sufficient to allow reasonably uniform load transfer intensities, to prevent large regions of separation, and yet to cover enough of the surface so as to prevent abrupt loading changes at the edge of contact. Another tool available to designers of joint replacement components is the use of compound structures, such as metallic trays supporting the polyethylene-bearing insert. For any particular application, a metallic tray stiffens the compound component, increasing the effective thickness. This causes the implant to act as if it had a decreased length-to-thickness ratio.

While the length-to-thickness ratio is a major determinant of the intensity of load transfer between the prosthesis and the cancellous bone bed, the area of coverage also plays an important role. For tibial plateaus, length-to-thickness ratio is a more important determinant than area of coverage for all conventionally designed prostheses. However, area of coverage can affect the intensity of the load transfer in an almost proportional manner (that is, 10 percent more area, 10 percent less stress). Good design principles therefore require maximizing the contact area within clinically accepted limitations.

Many of the early designs for cemented surface replacement prostheses incorporated central stems or peripheral pegs at the prosthesis–cancellous bone interface. These features provided mechanical interlocking to prevent sliding between contact surfaces at the time of implantation. Analytical studies later showed that these features have unexpected influences on load transfer (7). Centralized stems were thought to be a primary load transfer structure, but analysis demonstrated that because the stem is implanted in a region of low-density cancellous bone, 20 percent or less of the load is actually transferred by the stem. Nevertheless, the stem proves useful as a backup load transfer mechanism if soft-fibrous tissue develops under the edges of the tibial plateau. Tibial pegs, on the other hand, carry more load than might be expected. This is especially true for the pegs used to enhance fixation of porous ingrowth trays (8). When ingrowth occurs into the peg, a major portion of the load is transferred through the tray into regions surrounding the relatively high-stiffness peg–cancellous bone interface.

A common misconception with regard to load transfer between a surface replacement and an epiphyseal structure is that the implant has the ability to transfer load directly to the cortical shell. The cortical shell is very thin and flexible (9). Coupling at the circumference between implant and cortical shell, even if achievable, does not result in appreciable load transfer, since the shell stiffness differs little from the cancellous bone bed stiffness.

Load transfer devices have two major modes of mechanical failure, bone crushing at the prosthesis–cancellous bone interface and implant fracture. The failure process in the bone tissue occurs because of compressive overload and is usually a fatigue mode. Fatigue failure of bone is characterized clinically by repetitive loading, a gradual onset of pain, and bone resorption. The process may continue until gross resorption, subsidence, or dislocation occurs, or it may be self-limiting if the implant has another stable load transfer path available. We may reasonably expect bone to suffer compressive fatigue failure if the induced compressive stresses approach 60 to 80 percent of the yield stress (10). These stress levels may occur if the normal maximum compressive stresses in the cancellous bone of intact joints are increased by 50 to 100 percent due to the implantation of a surface replacement prosthesis. Factors that tend to increase the bone stresses are more flexible surface replacement components (a higher length-to-thickness ratio), a smaller surface area of joint loading (a lack of conformity under all loading conditions), edge load transfer of joint contact forces (resulting from either anteroposterior or medial-lateral instability), and features incorporating stress concentrators (peripheral pegs). Analyses have shown that the incorporation of a metallic tray can lessen the effects of load concentration and edge loading on the increased compressive stress at the prosthesis–cancellous bone interface (7). However, if extreme load concentration and edge loading can be avoided by other design means, compressive stresses at the surface of the cancellous bone can be kept well within tolerable limits by all-polyethylene tibial components.

The vast majority of load transfer components either are cemented or contain porous metallic surfaces that present opportunities for tissue ingrowth. Long-term viability of the cemented interface is a legitimate concern in clinical practice. The question is raised as to whether the cement interface can with-

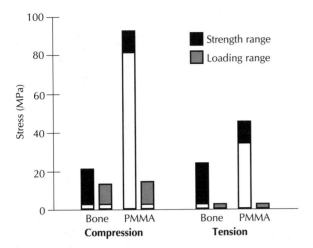

**Figure 7.11.** The maximum tensile and compressive stresses (yield stress) that PMMA cement and cancellous bone can tolerate are compared with the imposed stresses in these materials under the tibial plateau. Note that the fatigue strength is approximately 60 percent of the yield stress.

stand indefinite exposure to the loads at the interface between the prosthesis and the cancellous bone. We must first appreciate that the cement at the interface between prosthesis and bone is subjected to virtually the same stresses as the underlying bone tissue (7). The cement layer is typically thin, and PMMA cement has a modulus not substantially different from that of cancellous bone (Table 4.1 and Fig. 6.2).

Let's examine central plateau loading and edge loading for the knee joint illustrated in Figure 7.9A, and let's compare the stresses induced in the cancellous bone and in the cement with the yield and fatigue strengths of these two materials. In Figure 7.11 we show the tensile and compressive yield strengths of cancellous bone and of a typical bone cement. Superimposed upon these limits are the maximum stresses induced in the cancellous bone and in the cement by each of the two load configurations. As we previously stated, the stresses in the cement and in the cancellous bone are virtually the same. The peak stresses that we find in the cancellous bone are well below its fatigue strength (60 percent of its yield strength), even when all the load is placed centrally on one condyle. When the load is shifted to the edge of the condyle, the stress in the cancellous bone becomes critically close to its fatigue strength. This reinforces our previous conclusion that edge loading can lead to bone fatigue failure.

The situation with regard to bone cement is quite different. Neither concentrating the central load on a single condyle nor edge loading produces compressive stresses that approach the compressive fatigue strength of the cement. When we examine the maximum tensile stresses produced by these two loading conditions, we again see no likelihood of tensile fatigue failure based on the substantial difference between the induced tensile stress for these se-

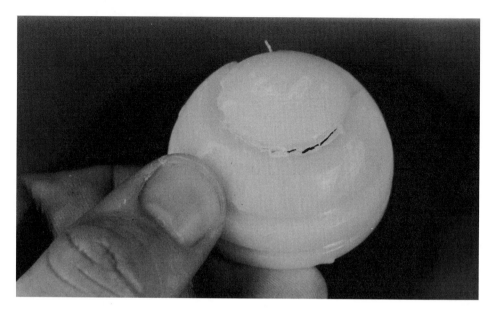

**Figure 7.12.** The fracture has propagated through the cup adjacent to a deep groove intended to enhance cement fixation.

vere loading conditions and the tensile fatigue strength. Thus, PMMA is an appropriately strong material to insert between the bone and prosthesis.

The second mode of failure experienced by load transfer surface replacements is fracture of the component. Failure almost always occurs because of fatigue, and both all-polyethylene components (11) and metal-backed polyethylene components (12) can suffer fatigue fracture. Acetabular cups are prone to polyethylene fatigue fracture in areas of stress concentration. The joint surface loading interacts with the contact forces at the prosthesis-bone interface to produce local bending in the acetabular cup. If the cup has deep grooves for cement interlock, local stresses in the polyethylene can exceed the polyethylene's fatigue limit, and gross failure can occur (Fig. 7.12).

Metallic trays sintered to enhance the bonding of a metallic porous coating lead to a reduction in fatigue strength. Sufficient bending moments are induced so that tensile stresses may exceed the reduced fatigue strength of the metal (Fig. 4.22). This is especially true if there are added stress concentrators, such as holes or sharp discontinuities at the junction of the central stem and the tray. For example, tibial plateaus intended to spare the posterior cruciate ligament have a posterior cutout that causes large local stresses. Stresses are caused by the distortion of the plateau when loads are placed posteriorly on the condyles. This effect is not strictly a stress concentration, but rather a structural weakening that results from the decreased torsional and bending stiffness of the tray. Fatigue cracks initiate in the high-stress regions near the corner of the cutout.

## CONTACT PROBLEMS IN TOTAL JOINT REPLACEMENT

While component fracture and mechanical failure at the prosthesis-bone interface are clinically important problems, these failure modes account for a minor fraction of all total joint failures. Typically, these mechanical failures occur within the first few years after implantation. The common long-term failure mode is surface wear. Failures from wear in a total joint replacement typically occur after 10 years and result from the creation and subsequent accumulation of polyethylene particulate debris in the joint's tissues. Since chemical degradation of the polyethylene material leads to increases in its elastic modulus and decreases in its failure properties, the chances of both wear failure (particulate debris formation) and mechanical failure are enhanced with time due to the high-stress environment. The latter problem is to some degree controllable by the design parameters.

Let's examine the influence of shape and material properties on the stresses induced in polyethylene components of total joint replacements. We will use two configurations of a finite element model (Fig. 7.13). The model represents a simple, all-polyethylene tibial plateau of the total condylar type. The posterior portion of the tibial plateau is loaded by the posterior portion of the femoral condyle. This represents a loading condition that would occur with the knee in flexion. In the second configuration, the tibial plateau is contacted more anteriorly with the distal portion of the femoral condyle, representing contact with the femoral component in extension. The compressive load across the knee during stair climbing will be assumed to be applied to one condyle. This represents normal loading conditions when a varus or valgus moment acts across the knee, producing a load of approximately four times body weight for the compressive joint reaction force at the knee ($4 \times 750$ newtons = 3000 newtons).

Our concern centers on the ability of the polyethylene to withstand the stresses that will be imposed upon it when the femoral component applies loads

**Figure 7.13.** The finite element model depicts an all-polyethylene tibial component. The model is constructed by dividing the component into elements, as shown for one section of the tibial plateau.

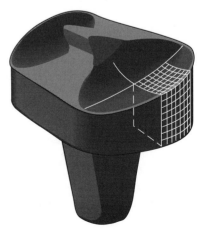

of up to 3000 newtons. We will compare the imposed stresses with the mechanical properties of the polyethylene material to determine the likelihood of failure. The method we choose to determine the stresses in polyethylene is finite element analysis. Unlike physical experiments, which can determine only contact pressures or surface strain, finite element methods can investigate stresses within the material. This will allow us to find the regions of highest stress and thus predict when and where failure will occur within the polyethylene component.

The model we will examine is constructed of a traditional rectangular array of small elements. Besides incorporating the geometry of the tibial component, the finite element model also contains appropriate material properties. By conducting tensile and compressive tests on ultra-high-molecular-weight polyethylene specimens, the stress-versus-strain behavior of the material can be characterized (Fig. 4.13). For simplicity in conducting the analysis, the actual curve can be approximated by the tangent method (Fig. 4.14). The original curve would be described as nonlinear. The tangent method produces a four-line approximation that would be described as "bilinear." This means that each quadrant (tensile or compressive loading) is represented by two straight lines.

Applying the finite element method of analysis involves deforming the polyethylene surface to conform to the shape of the metallic femoral component while producing a resistance to the compressive load equal to the joint reaction. Thus, the acceptable stress distribution produces a total contact force that is equal to the joint reaction and a pattern of deformation at the contact surface that results in a surface shape congruent to the femoral component.

Finite element analysis produces both stress distributions and displacement distributions throughout the entire tibial plateau. Typically, we direct our attention to the regions with the most intense stresses or the most severe displacements. In general, the most severe stresses occur directly on the contact surface. The finite element analysis shows a highly eccentric elliptical contact pattern for the position of extension (Fig. 7.14A) and a less eccentric elliptical contact pattern for the flexed position (Fig. 7.14B). The sign of the stress intensity indicates tension (+) or compression (−). The most intensive compressive stresses are at the center of the contact area, while the periphery shows modest tensile stresses. This phenomenon can be understood by realizing that the indentation caused by the contact displaces surface material most intensely at the center of contact—hence the high compression stresses. However, the contact surface is stretched in some regions to conform to the shape of the femoral component. The stretching is most severe at the periphery of the contact region—hence the tension stresses.

Loads on the knee joint are seldom applied statically. The knee is usually in motion when loaded. As we are aware, knee joint flexion and extension produce contact surfaces that move posteriorly with flexion and anteriorly with extension relative to the tibial plateau. Thus, over a typical loading cycle, such as

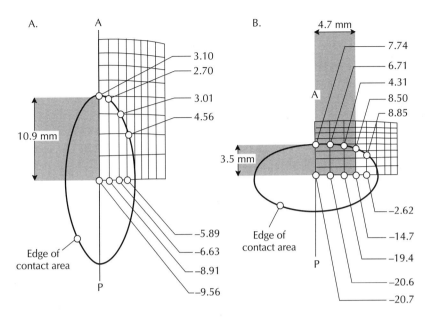

**Figure 7.14.** *A.* The contact area with the knee loaded in extension has central regions of compressive stress and peripheral regions of tensile stress. *B.* When loaded in the flexed position, the shape of the contact area changes with resultant increases in contact stress (13).

one step during stair climbing, the tibial plateau will experience a continuous sequence of different contact surfaces. Three such contact surfaces are shown in Figure 7.15 for the knee in transition from full extension to 75 degrees of flexion. A point on the component surface is in the center of the contact area at full extension, on the anterior edge of the contact area in partial flexion, and outside the region of contact at 75 degrees of flexion. The contact stresses experienced by this point in the polyethylene during one loading cycle are depicted in Figure 7.15. As the contact surface sweeps across the point, we note a transition from compressive stress to tensile stress, and finally a return to zero stress. This is a severe loading environment, which is conducive to fatigue failure. Unlike the hip joint, where the surface stresses on the polyethylene tend to remain compressive over the loading cycle, surface stresses on tibial plateaus experience reverse cycle (tension-compression-tension) loading.

Let's compare the intensity of the stresses in the tibial component with the material properties of the polyethylene (Fig. 4.13). We see that the compressive stresses produced in the center of the contact region take us beyond the linear region of the stress-versus-strain curve for polyethylene. Such high stresses can permanently deform the polyethylene and, if applied in sufficient numbers, can also induce fatigue damage. Thus, we see that the loading environment in a knee joint approaches the performance limit of ultra-high-molecular-weight polyethylene.

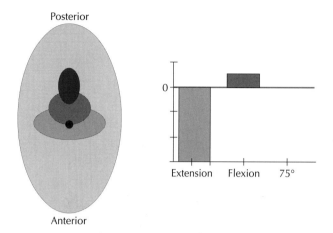

**Figure 7.15.** Three successive positions of the contact area corresponding to different degrees of flexion occupy different portions of the tibial plateau.

Since longevity of total joint replacements is of obvious concern, and since we recognize the relationship between the stress intensity at the contact surface and long-term surface degradation, we are naturally concerned about the relationship between the intensity of contact stresses and variables that can be controlled by design or by selection. Let's examine the effects of three design variables—component thickness, surface conformity, and the elastic modulus of the polyethylene material—on the contact stress intensity. These relationships are established by varying the appropriate parameter in the finite element model and re-solving the contact problem.

We will first examine the effects of component thickness for a total condylar knee joint that is loaded first in extension and then in flexion (Fig. 7.16). We notice the extreme nonlinearity of the results. For relatively thick components, of more than 8 millimeters, the maximum compressive contact stresses for a loading condition of 1500 newtons show little sensitivity to component thickness. Large increases in thickness, of as much as 50 percent (for example, from 8 millimeters to 12 millimeters), produce small changes in stress intensity (33 megapascals to 28 megapascals, or 15 percent). This is in direct contrast to the behavior of thinner tibial plateaus, where a 50 percent change in thickness (for example, from 8 millimeters to 4 millimeters) produces a 35 percent increase in contact stress. This illustrates the importance of choosing appropriately thick polyethylene components as a way of minimizing contact stress.

Conformity is another design variable that may be controlled or chosen. For a hip joint, clearance between the femoral and acetabular components can be controlled to produce a close conformity. Since both surfaces are spherical, articulation in all planes with close conformity is possible. For the knee joint, the surface may be described by the radii of curvature in the anteroposterior and medial-lateral planes. Since the curvature in the anteroposterior direction is dictated by the basic anatomy of the knee joint and by the requirement for full range of motion, the design choices are limited. Most design control can be exercised in the medial-lateral curvature. We will therefore examine the effect of conformity by varying the medial-lateral curvature of the joint components (Fig. 7.17). The changing radius represents variation of the medial-lateral curvature with anteroposterior curvature held constant. In general, the higher the mismatch in curvatures, the higher the contact stress. The minimum contact stress occurs when the radii of curvature are most conforming. For knee joints, this is not a practical solution, since high conformity of total condylar designs prevents axial rotation, a necessary kinematic feature of total knee prostheses. The surgeon must choose those contours that allow sufficient but restricted axial rotation, and that also have sufficient conformity to preclude unsatisfactorily high contact stresses.

To make this choice, we must first characterize the behavior of the joint surfaces that control axial rotation. Surfaces that have closely matching radii

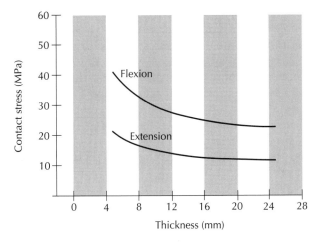

**Figure 7.16.** Contact stress plotted against thickness of the polyethylene component for the knee in flexion and extension.

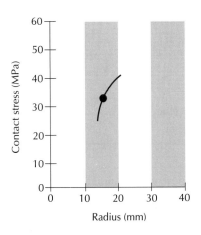

**Figure 7.17.** If all other radii are held constant, variations in the medial-lateral radius of the tibial plateau can greatly affect the contact stress.

of curvature (conforming surfaces) tend to resist rotation in the presence of compressive joint loads. This resistance to rotation is inversely proportional to the radius of curvature. Thus, flatter surfaces have less resistance to rotation. To choose the appropriate radius and conformity, analytical studies have produced a useful graphical tool (Fig. 7.18). On this plot of tibial medial-lateral radius of curvature versus femoral medial-lateral radius of curvature, two sets of lines are drawn. One set represents constant rotational resistance under joint compressive load, and one set represents constant maximum contact stress. By choosing the desired rotational resistance, the radii with the least contact stress can be selected.

With presently available materials, neither designer nor surgeon has much control over the elastic modulus for the bearing material in total joint replacements. Currently available total joints have one bearing surface composed of a high-elastic-modulus metallic alloy and a mating surface composed of relatively low-elastic-modulus polyethylene. Because the modulus of a metal such as cobalt alloy is approximately 200 times that of polyethylene (Table 4.1), the stresses induced by contact loads are essentially controlled by the modulus of the polyethylene component. Mechanical properties of polyethylene can be altered so that the modulus ranges from approximately 1 to 2 gigapascals. For the contours usually encountered in total joint replacements, this modulus range produces contact stress variations somewhat greater than 1 to 2. Available polyethylene formulations show strong association between the strength of the polyethylene and its elastic modulus. However, increasing the material's strength and hence its elastic modulus carries with it the penalty of increasing contact stress. Careful analysis is required to determine if the increase in con-

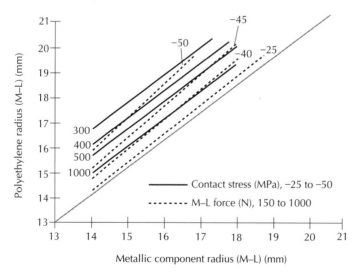

**Figure 7.18.** The applied load was 3000 newtons. The anteroposterior radii corresponded to those for a knee in extension. The polyethylene thickness was 7 millimeters; the medial-lateral displacement was 0.25 millimeters. *(Courtesy of Donald Bartel, Ph.D.)*

tact stress due to higher modulus overshadows the inherent strength advantage of the enhanced, higher-modulus polyethylene.

Polyethylene properties may be deliberately changed by subjecting the material to controlled conditions of elevated temperature and pressure. Unfortunately, other conditions also alter the properties of polyethylene. Most notable among these conditions are radiation sterilization and exposure to oxidative environments. These conditions can decrease the molecular chain length and increase cross-linking between chains. These alterations result in an increase in density and elastic modulus. The increase in modulus results in higher contact stresses.

Total joint replacements have been in clinical use for almost three decades. It is becoming apparent that one of the major concerns associated with this technology is the wear life of the prosthetic components. Clinical experience with total hip joints shows that with appreciable wear polyethylene acetabular components can require revision as early as the second decade after implantation. Reports of the experience with several total knee designs show that wear may be a limiting factor before the end of the first decade, while others last well into the second decade. Whereas the contact surface geometries in total hip prostheses may be universally described as spherical, the geometry of the contact surfaces of total knee prostheses vary widely. Different contact surface geometries are associated with different contact stresses; hence, wear rates for total knee prostheses will show design-to-design variations that are considerably greater than those for total hip prostheses.

Wear rates for total hip prostheses are controlled by the contact stresses. These, in turn, are controlled by the joint geometry, its material properties, and the joint compressive load. For the hip joint, the contact geometry does not change appreciably throughout the entire functional range of motion. Conformity is high throughout the entire range of motion. The corresponding contact stresses are low, and the polyethylene wears by production of microscopic free-surface particles. This is in contrast to total knee prostheses, which have relatively nonconforming surfaces. The contact stresses at the surface are considerably higher than for total hip prostheses. Microscopic wear particles are produced, but in addition, the larger stresses cause surface and subsurface fractures that result in the liberation of larger particulate debris.

### *References*

1. Woo SL-Y, Lothringer KS, Akeson WH, Coutts RD, Woo YK, Simon BR, Gomez MA. Less rigid internal fixation plates: Historical perspectives and new concepts. J Orthop Res 1984;1:431-449.

2. Rybicki EF, Simonen FA, Mills EJ, Hassler CR, Scoles P, Milne D, Weis EB. Mathematical and experimental studies on the mechanics of plated transverse fractures. J Biomech 1974;7:377-384.

3. Cheal EJ, Hayes WC, White AA III, Perren SM. Three-dimensional finite element analysis of a simplified compression plate fixation system. J Biomech Eng 1984; 106:295-301.

4. Crowninshield RD, Brand RA, Johnston RC, Pedersen DR. An analysis of femoral prosthesis design: The effects on proximal femur loading. In: Salvati EA, ed. The hip. St. Louis: CV Mosby, 1981:111-122.

5. Rimnac CM, Wright TM, Bartel DL, Burstein AH. Failure analysis of a total femoral component: A fracture mechanics approach. In: Hudson CM, Rich TP, eds. Case histories involving fatigue and fracture mechanics. Philadelphia: ASTM, 1986: 377-388.

6. Bartel DL, Burstein AH, Toda MD, Edwards DL. The effect of conformity and plastic thickness on contact stresses in metal-backed plastic implants. J Biomech Eng 1985;107:193-199.

7. Bartel DL, Burstein AH, Santavicca EA, Insall JN. Performance of the tibial component in total knee replacement: Conventional and revision designs. J Bone Joint Surg 1982;64A:1026-1033.

8. Dawson JM, Bartel DL. Consequences of an interference fit on the fixation of porous-coated tibial components in total knee replacement. J Bone Joint Surg 1992; 74A:233-238.

9. Lotz JC, Gerhart TN, Hayes WC. Mechanical properties of metaphyseal bone in the proximal femur. J Biomech 1991;24:317-329.

10. Choi K, Goldstein SA. A comparison of the fatigue behavior of human trabecular and cortical bone tissue. J Biomech 1992;25:1371-1381.

11. Salvati EA, Wright TM, Burstein AH, Jacobs B. Fracture of polyethylene acetabular cups. J Bone Joint Surg 1979;61A:1239-1242.

12. Ranawat CS, Johanson NA, Rimnac CM, Wright TM, Schwartz RE. Retrieval analysis of porous-coated components for total knee replacement: A report of two cases. Clin Orthop 1986;209:244-248.

13. Bartel DL, Bicknell VL, Wright TM. The effect of conformity, thickness, and material on stresses in ultra-high molecular weight components for total joint replacement. J Bone Joint Surg 1986;68A:1041-1051.

# INDEX

Page numbers in *italics* denote figures; those followed by "t" denote tables.

219